P9-CBI-225

THROUGH THE VALLEY OF SHADOWS

THROUGH THE VALLEY
OF SHADOWS

Living Wills, Intensive Care, and Making
Medicine Human

Samuel Morris Brown

OXFORD
UNIVERSITY PRESS

OXFORD
UNIVERSITY PRESS

Oxford University Press is a department of the University of Oxford. It furthers
the University's objective of excellence in research, scholarship, and education
by publishing worldwide. Oxford is a registered trade mark of Oxford University
Press in the UK and certain other countries.

Published in the United States of America by Oxford University Press
198 Madison Avenue, New York, NY 10016, United States of America.

© Oxford University Press 2016

First Edition published in 2016

Library of Congress Cataloging-in-Publication Data
Brown, Samuel Morris, author.
Through the valley of shadows : living wills, intensive care, and making medicine
human / Samuel Morris Brown.
p. ; cm.
Includes index.
ISBN 978-0-19-939295-7 (hardcover : alk. paper) — ISBN 978-0-19-939296-4
(Ebook (UPDF)) — ISBN 978-0-19-939297-1 (Ebook (EPUB))
I. Title.
[DNLM: 1. Living Wills—ethics. 2. Attitude to Death. 3. Intensive Care—
psychology. 4. Patient Participation. 5. Right to Die—ethics. W 85.5]
R726.8
179.7—dc23
2015032315

1 3 5 7 9 8 6 4 2

Printed by Sheridan, USA

CONTENTS

SECTION TWO
PRESENT

CONTENTS

ACKNOWLEDGMENTS

I am indebted to those who have paved the way for me in this endeavor. Michael Howell and Barbara Sarnoff-Lee had the vision to establish a profoundly patient-centered system in the intensive care units (ICUs) of Beth Israel-Deaconess Medical Center in Boston. They have trained me how to formally incorporate the insights and experiences of patients and families. Others with no academic training have tutored me even more. With courage and grace, sometimes distracted and horrified by the ways their bodies have betrayed them, my patients and their families have allowed me to care for them as an ICU physician over the years. They have demanded, sometimes vocally, often implicitly, that I bring to them both the best of my technical skill and all of my human self. These excellent people have accompanied me throughout my journey.

All patient vignettes have been disguised and/or hybridized to maintain confidentiality, unless otherwise noted. Vignettes that are extensively hybridized are noted as such in the endnotes.

I thank the Division of Medical Ethics and Humanities at the University of Utah, an excellent group of scholars and friends to whom I owe a great deal. The Division also supported the work of my able research assistant, Linda Carr-Lee Faix.

Intermountain Healthcare is a wonderful place to work. People are eager, collegial, and committed to their work, and there is an institutional commitment to understanding and delivering the highest quality medical care possible. My colleagues within the Center for Humanizing Critical Care deserve my deep gratitude, as do the other clinicians and researchers who strive daily to make ICUs safer and better for patients and families.

I dedicate this book to my wife, Kate Holbrook. She fills the world with meaning and my soul with light. Our walk together through the valley of shadows has wrenched and rebuilt me, and while I would never wish cancer on anyone, I am grateful for who we are becoming in its aftermath.

I thank Sarah Beesley, Zackary Sholem Berger, Spencer Brown, Linda Carr-Lee Faix, Peter Crompton, Susan Hamilton, Debra Hampton, Ramona Hopkins, Jana Riess, Richard Rigby, Brett Rushforth, and Jacob Stegenga for reading and providing feedback on the manuscript at various stages of its development. I thank my agent Lisa Adams for her incredible ear for prose and her capacity to see a book within the barest of confused scratches on paper. And I thank Peter Ohlin and his associates at Oxford University Press for shepherding this project from proposal to published book with wisdom, insight, and enthusiasm.

Introduction

John looked exhausted, almost penitent. Bright red blood trickled from his mouth. A giant ulcer near the top of his small intestine was bleeding briskly despite attempts to control the hemorrhage through a flexible scope. We needed to take over his breathing in order to stop the bleeding surgically. As the attending physician caring for John, I felt the adrenaline surge of an acute crisis. Because intubating—placing a breathing tube through a patient's mouth and into the windpipe—through a mouthful of blood is difficult, the procedure requires extreme focus. Absorbed by the task at hand, I saw only John's airway and the equipment I would use to perform the intubation. Choking back tears as John became sleepier, his wife Kathy suddenly yelled toward me, "He is not DNR! You can't let him die!"

Her announcement surprised me: It would not have occurred to me to refuse to resuscitate a healthy man in his midsixties, so I had not even checked his "code status" in the medical chart to see whether it included a "Do Not Resuscitate" (DNR) order forbidding certain treatments during a medical crisis. An order to not resuscitate often makes sense near the end of a person's life, but by all accounts John had been hale and hearty before this episode of treatable but life-threatening bleeding. As we rushed to intubate John and administer a massive transfusion of blood, I told Kathy that any DNR order wouldn't interfere with our full efforts for his recovery, even if his heart were to stop. I felt her fear and anxiety deep in my stomach, where it merged with my preparation for the intubation procedure.

The intubation went well, and we got John safely to the operating room. During surgery, Kathy and I found time to speak at length in John's empty room in the intensive care unit (ICU). I reassured her that despite the dramatic bleeding, John's prospects looked reasonable over-all, and she slowly regained her composure. Still bothered by the DNR order in John's chart, she explained, "He was just trying to tell people that he didn't want to be a vegetable. He didn't mean anything more than that." It was hard enough to see John nearly drowning in blood; it almost broke Kathy's heart to have to correct a misleading legal state-ment in the midst of that health crisis.

My medical team was proud of the careful work they had done to stop the bleeding and save John's life, but we had missed the psychologi-cal harm that the system had inadvertently done to Kathy and John. She had fully expected that we would refuse to save his life on the basis of his DNR order. That possibility hadn't even crossed our minds until Kathy's tearful plea brought it to our attention.

People require treatment in the ICU for many different reasons—strokes, motorcycle accidents, blood clots in the lungs, internal bleed-ing, infected gall bladders, drug overdoses—what unites almost all of them is a high risk of death without treatment. Sometimes an ICU admission comes when death is already imminent, perhaps from wide-spread, advanced cancer. Sometimes people with serious but manage-able illnesses like chronic kidney failure experience a temporary crisis, and sometimes a life-threatening infection strikes a previously healthy person. Many ICU patients now survive, while some die either during or shortly after their stay in the ICU. Some benefit greatly from their time in the ICU, while others would never have wanted to be admitted there in the first place. Every person coming through the ICU has specific, individual needs; no single approach to caring for them will work.

While in John's case we were at risk for providing too little treatment, in many cases we risk providing too much medical treatment in the ICU. Stories abound about people whose chances for a quiet and dignified passage from life drown in a turbulent sea of carelessly applied medical technology. I have personally witnessed many such painful dramas.

Barry's story ran differently from John's. Barry had been dying of emphysema for five months when I met him on his return to the ICU from a nursing home. He had been bedridden for so long that despite everyone's best attempts to reposition him every hour, his tailbone protruded through the skin of his backside, a misery that caused deep infection. The bacteria in his bone had spread to his blood, and he was returning to the hospital with septic shock. A tracheostomy kept him alive but prevented speech. By the time I cared for him, he never tried to speak anymore, and no one could tell whether it was because he was too tired or he had suffered permanent brain damage from one of his cardiac arrests. Everyone had been reluctant to confront the possibility of death early in his hospitalization, and now it seemed too late for such conversations, as he slowly worsened amid transfers from nursing homes to ICUs and back.

Cases like Barry's haunt us clinicians, and we often numb the pain by expressing our technical proficiency at operating life support systems or by looking for shortcuts to get us out of difficult conversations. Throughout this book, I will tell the twin stories of how we as human beings experience life-threatening illness and how the current medical system fails us in our time of need, a failure driven by clinicians' inability to see the world the way patients and families do.

As an ICU physician and medical professor, I did not originally appreciate how many needless stresses are imposed on patients and families as side effects of the amazing and strenuous work of intensive care. What does it matter if there are some communication failures, I used to think, as long as we save people from death? I was saving lives; I couldn't also be a social worker. But the system was broken, I was complicit, and we were harming patients and families in myriad ways.

I never meant to be callous. I tried not to be. But I was distracted by the urgency of running life support systems, by the number of patients in the ICU, and by the complexity of their medical problems. Stress and distraction led to failures to communicate with or acknowledge my patients as human beings. Such failures were so common that they seemed the inevitable result of external forces. What appears inescapable often seems not worth the effort to fix it.

Like many of my colleagues, I chose the field of intensive care because I loved the drama of struggling against disease and physical crisis and because I wanted to save lives. The work we do is heady stuff. Even the name of my specialty, "critical care medicine," emphasizes the idea that everything hangs in the balance. A skeptic might wonder whether we are just trying to reassure ourselves that we are important. Without our *critical* work, disease would win. Consistent with this framing, we ICU clinicians are sometimes prone to do rather than think.

Acting instead of reflecting made me feel like I mattered, as if I were doing battle with the diseases that threatened my patients' lives. The military metaphors that we physicians are sometimes accused of using—we go to battle with death—exist for a reason. These metaphors allow us to survive the terrible stresses of training and then medical practice, and they add a moral substance to our lives. But there are risks to these metaphors; they can lead to a kind of blindness.

In retrospect I am a bit surprised at how long it took me to realize that something was deeply wrong with the medical system in which I worked. The blinders I wore are even more striking in light of my work on intellectual history. When I was in college I couldn't decide between studying the history of religion and going to medical school. I spent a year or two vacillating between the two career choices. Ultimately I felt that I would see most clearly as a physician but still kept one eye on religion and culture. During my residency, I realized I could vent some emotional steam by researching and writing cultural history. The past was a safe place for me to ask big questions. While writing a book about death culture and American religion before the Civil War, I read hundreds of accounts of the "good death." I began to wonder why good dying was incredibly rare in the hospitals where I practiced medicine. That would make an interesting project someday, I thought. Someday.

In 2012, my wife, herself a religious historian, told me one Sunday night in August that her vision had become blurry, but she had ignored the hazy vision because she was chairing a conference on women and religion. I assumed she'd had a small blood clot in her eye, maybe a retinal detachment, some minor medical problem to prove that we were entering middle age. Instead, the eye doctors found a large melanoma lifting her retina off the back of her eye. The kindest of the doctors told me over the phone that he thought Kate probably had just a year or two to live. Kate and I cried together in the guest room in our basement, far from the curious gaze of our three young children. The sobbing felt like a seizure, convulsions of grief that robbed us of speech. A long and painful process followed, concluding with a prosthetic eye and excellent prospects of survival.

Through Kate's melanoma, I experienced firsthand the utter inability of our current medical system to support people during life-threatening illness. Our system wields medical technology with astonishing skill but does almost nothing to help people make medical decisions or weather life-threatening illness emotionally and spiritually. While we were grateful for the chance for cure that surgical removal of her eye provided, we felt wounded needlessly by the system and the clinicians who were its accidental accomplices. As my mind slowly cleared from the misery of Kate's diagnosis and operations, we settled back into a new way of living. I came to understand my professional obligations in a new light.

Kate's illness persuaded me to pull together the various elements of my career in order to attend carefully to the human side of life-threatening illness. I realized in the clarity that sometimes accompanies crisis that to fix these problems would require my knowledge of statistics and clinical research, my expertise in history, and my years at the bedside treating patients with life-threatening illness. In order to accomplish this task, I expanded the scope of my medical research, founded the Center for Humanizing Critical Care at Intermountain Healthcare, and wrote this book.

Millions of patients and families who pass through modern ICUs every year receive generally high quality medical care but are utterly and even cruelly unsupported as human beings. As they walk through what I have come to see as the valley of shadows—a strange world stretching between life and death, filled with ominous darkness and misapprehended threats but also the desperate hope for human meaning in the face of possible death—they are left without guides, abandoned to make their way alone through these medical precincts of mortality. The majority of patients and families come out of the ICU with post-traumatic stress, anxiety, or depression. They are more shell-shocked than combat veterans, according to an array of recent studies. And those are the survivors. The people who do not survive are not only dead; the medical system has often stolen from them the chance to complete their lives meaningfully, distorting their final days in an explosion of medical technology. We health professionals may have deformed their deaths, in the phrase of the medical ethicist Daniel Callahan.[1] Some of these terrible outcomes are unavoidable, but many are inflicted needlessly. It doesn't have to be this way. Those who survive deserve better from us, and so do those who die.

Two basic facts about patients arriving in the ICU must be acknowledged: They are human beings, and we cannot predict their fate with certainty. Because patients in the ICU are human beings, they and their families deserve a strategy for care that incorporates physiological and psychological insights within the context of humane treatment. Because none of us can predict the future with certainty, they and their families need a medical system that will serve them well regardless of whether they survive their ICU stay, one that will work with them at every point on the issues that matter most to them. Living and dying are dynamic processes. The contexts and conditions change frequently, often unpredictably. Solutions to these problems must be true to the dynamic nature of life and, when the time comes, death.

The fact of our uncertainty about ultimate outcomes creates an interdependence among patients and healthcare professionals that sometimes feels burdensome to clinicians but can instead be beautiful. We clinicians do not know at the moment we provide them whether our treatments will succeed. While physicians' historical tendency to overtreat dying patients is well known, often they swing to the other side. It's difficult for clinicians to try to save a patient who ultimately dies; it takes a heavy emotional toll to hope for survival and then be disappointed. Unless clinicians are able to make sense of that burden, a kind of nihilism can harm both them and their patients. They may be inclined not to treat patients who are at significant risk for death, even when the patients would have wanted treatment. One way through this difficulty—if we are to honor patients and provide the care they actually desire, we will have to treat many patients who do not survive—is to acknowledge an interconnection among patients and with ourselves. We clinicians can consecrate the sadness we feel when a patient dies despite our best efforts as part of the offering we make on behalf of those who survive. By understanding my sadness at the death of patients as a kind of sacred offering, I have found myself better able to support both those who survive and those who die.

Clinicians' responses to life-threatening illness have been such a mess for so long that a host of partially effective or basically ineffective solutions have been proposed. I do not discuss them all in this book. The most persistent of the solutions has been a collection of legal documents called "advance directives." They are "advance" because they are intended to represent decisions made *before* they apply in real life. They are "directives" because they are meant to contain instructions for medical professionals. These legal documents have become culturally influential; in much of polite society, having one has become a duty, like wearing a seatbelt or buying life insurance. The goal of these documents is noble: to ensure that an individual's voice is heard even when she is unconscious. But these documents have for the most part been either ineffective or actively counterproductive. Instead of meaningful guidance through the valley of shadows, these documents have furthered an approach that often diminishes rather than enhances patients and their families during life-threatening illness.

The advance directives represent the fruits of a system that critics call "disclosurism," the notion that providing complicated legal documents to people protects them from exploitation by corporations or government agencies. As critics have noted, the legal documents that disclosurism creates do more for large corporations than they do for the people interacting with them. Private individuals are generally left disoriented and unsure of what they have just agreed to. The same is often true of advance directives, just as it was for John and Kathy.

We often don't know what to do when life is threatened. Hazard lurks on both sides. We are like the ancient Greek sailors steering their boats between Scylla and Charybdis. On the one side stands the arrogant paternalism that had physicians treating patients and families like toddlers, robbing them of choice and dignity. On the other side stands the disclosurism that offers only the appearance of autonomy. Between them lies the soulful and healthful path that I point out in this book. Both the paternalism of medicine through the 1960s and the advance directive paradigm that replaced it have failed us as human beings. The human path, the one that we are called to walk, is the middle way between the Scylla of paternalism and the Charybdis of bare autonomism. That middle way can create meaning and sustain community in the face of our mortality, walking through the valley of shadows together in deep and mutual commitment.

Advance directives run the gamut. They started out as "living wills" in 1969. These documents allowed patients to refuse certain medical treatments if they were unconscious. In parallel came "code status" determinations, by which patients could refuse or allow life support treatments if their hearts stopped. More recently, detailed documents place precise limits on the types of medical therapies that physicians can provide in the event of specific medical catastrophes.

Advance directives have serious defects, especially the assumptions they make about autonomy and the way the human mind works. In the following chapters, I discuss the troubles with advance directives and the problems they are intended to solve at some length. Here, I highlight several of the central problems in the stories of three patients and their families: Stacy, Christopher, and Tyler.

Stacy Hill[2] was a vivacious thirty-six-year-old professional mountain climber. On a technical climb in a canyon near Salt Lake City, her safety anchors failed during a minor fall, and a sharp edge of granite struck her, hard, just below the base of her skull. The LifeFlight evacuation team got her off the mountain quickly enough that she survived into the care of our trauma surgeons. Stacy slowly awakened in our ICU to discover that she had a high spinal cord injury and was unable to move her arms or legs. She had broken her neck, though her wits were mostly intact. A friend and fellow climber had been disabled by paralysis from a spinal cord injury, so Stacy had thought about what life would be like if the same thing ever happened to her. She had once told her husband, Joe, that she couldn't conceive of life without rock climbing, let alone as a quadriplegic. In the ICU, she began to mouth words to Joe and her family that they understood as consistent with her prior opinion. "Die," seemed to be the message her lips traced around the plastic breathing tube, although no one could be sure how alert she actually was or how to interpret what she was silently mouthing.

Stacy's brother, Steve, was a nurse in the emergency room (ER) and ICU in their small hometown hospital in western Colorado. He too had heard Stacy say that she would never want to live if she were stuck in a wheelchair. Steve was Stacy's most ardent spokesman, and he lobbied strongly for the medical team to honor his sister's wishes. He even threatened a lawsuit if the doctors failed to honor her requests. He had seen too many miserable deaths in his career as a nurse to let them keep his sister alive against her will.

After three days of Steve's increasingly angry insistence and Stacy's earnest if inarticulate pleading, the medical team was close to stopping treatment. No one wanted to be cruel, and the doctors half-feared a lawsuit. But the medical team felt queasy about letting Stacy die. So the senior physician requested an ethics consultation, and the ethics committee refused to obey Steve's request on the grounds that Stacy would soon be able to communicate her wishes clearly. The disagreement with the medical team finally escalated to lawyers and judges. By the time the litigation started that next week, Stacy had awakened more and grown accustomed to the ventilator. She was no longer choking on the breathing tube. Joe began to resist Steve's opinions and was able to talk more with Stacy, who was much calmer than she had been. The team located an assistive computer tablet that allowed Stacy to communicate by looking at letters on the screen. She started asking questions about life with paralysis. It took a few days of pondering and communicating with Stacy, but Joe and Stacy finally overruled Steve, and Stacy survived the crisis. While her life was never the same, over time she settled into life with disability and later coached other people who had survived spinal cord injury.

In part, the near disaster with Stacy was due to her brother's moral distress and his failure to anticipate that Stacy would adapt to her disability. Like many healthcare workers—especially nurses, according to several studies—Steve had been burned often enough by treating patients who later died or otherwise suffered under his watch that he had come to find life support distasteful. Disability stigma, the intuitive revulsion most people feel when trying to imagine life with disability, probably also played a role. The fear of his sister's paralysis and his own moral distress about life support therapy may have combined with his earnest desire to honor her wishes to make Steve think that stopping life-prolonging treatments was the right thing.

While moral distress may have propelled him, Steve's stated reason for his request to remove the ventilator focused on an interpretation of Stacy's autonomy. Autonomy is one of the founding tenets of Western bioethics; it is the notion that we are obligated to respect each individual's capacity to govern herself or be directed by values and considerations that are chosen internally rather than imposed externally. The opposite of oppression, autonomy draws on deep roots in our culture. In medicine, autonomy generally has been considered in terms of an individual's right to refuse procedures.

In theory, autonomy is a wonderful thing, and it is a crucial goal in life and in medicine. In practice, though, the way autonomy is implemented in contemporary America—and the living wills that are among the flagship products of contemporary medical autonomy—can, paradoxically, diminish the autonomy they hope to preserve. In Stacy's case, a superficial autonomy, based on blind spots and understandable impatience with the miseries of the ICU, interfered with the deep expression of her autonomy. The trick was to carry her from an acute threat into a new life so that she could decide whether she, with time to understand the actual decision at hand, desired that new life to continue.[3]

We all will speculate about future states of disability in our own ways. Those different ways are part of how we experience life as individuals. Temporary rejection of new disability is so common that it would be incautious to assume that it represents a considered opinion. There will be patients whose lives are already wrapping up for whom the further misery of an injury will signal that it's time to allow death to come. But for many people, some time and reflection so often lead to a change of opinion that we should not rush to "honor" a transient, hypothetical claim about what life has to look like.

An authentic autonomy, one true to the individual's actual values and priorities, is best protected when clinicians practice what the psychiatrist and ethicist Jodi Halpern has called empathy. To describe their sense of an autonomy that is more than trivial or superficial, others have described "dialogic" or "psychological" autonomy; some legal theorists describe a "soft" paternalism that is justified to preserve such autonomy. I think of the process of allowing individuals to direct their lives in ways that are authentic to them as human beings as a kind of guidance. Whatever this autonomy is called, it is often lost in advance directives, in part because they fail to appreciate the "predictably irrational" (in Dan Ariely's phrase) ways we all process information, especially during a health crisis.

In Stacy's case, one such predictable irrationality nearly led to her death. As we will see in chapter 4, we human beings are terrible at imagining our future selves accurately. Stacy (and Steve) couldn't see how Stacy would adapt to her new life with paralysis. Treating her prior conversation as a firm directive demanded that she and her family commit to just such a faulty prediction, without new information from Stacy herself.

The distress that drove Steve to request his sister's death is understandable. It's common among healthcare workers. Clinicians often experience complicated, troubled feelings about the treatments they provide. ICU physicians do things that would qualify as torture if they were performed with any other goal than prolonging life with the individual's consent. Not to put too fine a point on it, but we tie people to a bed when necessary for their safety, inject them with mind-altering drugs, and shove tubes down their throats and into most of their other orifices.

We clinicians generally think that what we do provides an important service and makes the world a better place. We believe that our labors carry the promise of patients healed and lives saved. When it doesn't seem that our labors are likely to bear the fruit we hope for, we have a tendency to transition rapidly to the opposite extreme of not wanting anything done. It's too painful to see oneself torturing a person for no clear benefit.

Researchers describe those negative feelings as moral distress and describe a false sense of identity with patients as "pseudo empathy," in opposition to true empathy. The horror that brutal treatments might be endured in vain stands behind the reality that in most ICUs there are two settings: "do everything" and "do nothing."

Both "do everything" and "do nothing" cause problems. The "do everything" mentality has deformed the deaths of thousands of individuals and devastated many others. But "do nothing" may lead to needless death that fails to honor an individual in her human richness.

Moral distress partly explains why my partners recommended to Christopher's family that they take him off the ventilator and let nature take its course after he had been ill for several weeks with swine flu and still showed no signs of improvement. The H1N1 influenza pandemic in early 2009 was a miserable time for all of us. It felt like every day we came in to work to find another young person struggling for life on the ventilator. When the occasional patient with H1N1 appears in the ICU still, we all shiver a little with the memory of those miserable days before the vaccine was available.

My partners had carried Christopher through the most difficult phases of the influenza, when his life hung in the balance with each troubled breath on the ventilator. But, four weeks after his lungs had clearly begun to heal, he remained comatose. The staff lost hope in his eventual recovery. He appeared to be in a vegetative state, and it was not clear why. Yet that uncertainty didn't stop the team from moving from "do everything" to "do nothing."

Resisting the treating team, Christopher's family dug in their heels. He was too young—all of forty-three—and he hadn't had an obvious reason to lose higher brain function other than the terrible influenza and the sedatives that had been required to keep him calm on the ventilator. My partners pressed on. After nine weeks in the ICU, Christopher and his family moved to a skilled nursing facility, which we expected would be his permanent home. We were all stunned, embarrassed, and delighted to hear that he had awakened about a month later. In retrospect, Christopher's brain had just been hibernating.

Christopher's case exemplifies how difficult prediction is. It's not just patients or families who often get it wrong; it's the whole enterprise of predicting the future. This is true even when specialists are the ones making the predictions. All too often physicians and nurses are simply unable to foresee patients' outcomes accurately. Christopher and many patients like him remind us of the tentative nature of most of our forecasts. In the face of inevitable uncertainty, clinicians may unconsciously allow their distaste for painful treatments to cloud their judgment in ways that sap patients of their autonomy.

Decisions about treatment predominated in the stories of Stacy and Christopher and are central to the advance directives paradigm. But that focus on decisions has tended to give short shrift to the pressing needs of patients and families in the ICU. We don't have much insight about what to do during desperate situations that will ultimately turn out okay, or how to deal with the inherent uncertainty that accompanies providing care to people on the brink of death. How do we avoid causing needless psychological harm to people who have to make their way through the valley of the shadow of death? Because mortality looms so large in those situations, it's easy for us clinicians to forget about the damage we inadvertently do to survivors and their families.

Everybody in the ICU took care of Tyler at some point. He had terrible liver failure from autoimmune hepatitis, a condition in which his immune system treated his liver as a foreign invader. He spent several months in the ICU, most of it on a ventilator, while he awaited a liver transplant. Unless you've lived with cirrhosis, it's tough to understand just how wrenching the final stages of liver failure are. Tyler's wife, Audrey, stood at the side of his bed for several hours a day through those months. She managed to keep a stiff upper lip through all the dramas of his terrible disease. And there was plenty of drama. At various times, his lungs flooded with blood, his kidneys shut down, and he lapsed into a deep coma. During each setback he looked perilously ill, but even though we were fighting an uphill battle, he still had reasonable chances for survival.

Once, though, Tyler's situation looked grim: at best a 5 percent chance of recovery. He was in his deepest coma yet, blood clots and bruises scattered throughout his brain (a consequence of the leakiness of brain capillaries when liver failure is at its worst), and he was in seizures that we could not stop despite trying all available seizure medications. I wasn't quite sure how to tell Audrey that I was becoming pessimistic. We'd been through so much already, and I saw her courage in the face of terror with each setback. I did not want to steal that courage from her, but I also did not want to sugar coat my way into a lie. I'd been honest with her about Tyler's chances all along, and I had also communicated my cautious optimism. So we sat down, and I talked about how committed I was to giving Tyler every possible chance for survival. I also described how worried I had become. She looked horrified and dispirited. I returned a couple of hours later and apologized. I told her that I wondered whether I should have held onto that worry for her, that it might be my job to carry the emotional stress of life-threatening illness on her behalf. Through a tired smile she told me that she preferred the whole truth, even when it was painful.

In any event, Tyler's seizures calmed enough after a week that the surgeons were willing to transplant his liver. (The transplant surgeons normally reserve the limited number of donor organs for people who they believe will recover after the transplant operation.) It wasn't quick, and it wasn't easy, but Tyler ultimately recovered. We all get misty-eyed whenever he stops by the ICU to say hello in his blue baseball cap. Mixed with that giddy pleasure at his recovery, though, is worry over whether we took care of Audrey the way we should have. I suspect that she bears needless scars from her ICU experience. If so, she's one of many ICU veterans with similar scars.

Audrey's and Tyler's story emphasizes the importance of personalized support for families even when there is no decision to be made. The razor-sharp focus on individual patients has tended to blind clinicians to the needs of the loved ones who accompany patients through the ICU. The medical system often forgets that autonomy is enmeshed in networks of relationship and human belonging. Especially as we walk through the valley of shadows, we are not and should not be alone. Whether we are patient or family, we need a guide who is flexible and appropriate to our individual needs, not a simplistic list of requirements for when we should be allowed to die. We need relevant, tailored guidance through the valley of shadows, not an idiosyncratic insurance policy in the form of a living will. Such "insurance policies" do little to serve individuals who may choose to die rather than live in a disabled state, or people who would choose to continue to live with disability after an adjustment period.

I've often run over that conversation with Audrey in my mind. Was I being pessimistic or realistic? What could I have done better? Was it right to tell her just how worried I was? I had no training, no evidence to go by, and no reliable scientific literature to guide me through that encounter. What was the best way to accompany Audrey and Tyler on their frightening journey?

Communication is not just an extra duty that especially attentive doctors take on. Communication is the sine qua non of authentic autonomy. Without careful, effective communication, decisions cannot actually reflect the choices the individual hopes to make. Yet the model of autonomy that healthcare workers commonly apply during life-threatening illness is prone to inauthenticity, as we run through permissions for a brief list of dramatic medical procedures, rather than addressing patients' and families' experiences, values, and priorities. The situations in the ICU are overwhelming, and stated preferences may be driven by desperate confusion or reflect prior speculations not grounded in reality.

Attempted suicide may be one of the hardest areas to work through because questions of autonomy are particularly murky then. The requests to stop treatment that I receive after attempted suicide generally involve loving family members with deeply conflicted feelings. Maria asked me, after her troubled daughter Diane had attempted to end her struggles with diabetes with an intentional insulin overdose, whether we could just let nature take its course. "Can't we just let her go?" she asked. These are some of the most painful conversations I have. I feel deep sympathy for the loved ones, knowing how miserable life has been for everyone involved and what a struggle awaits them after recovery. But I remember well the studies showing that only about one in ten survivors of a suicide attempt will go on to die by their own hand.[4] As a general rule, a suicide attempt is not an expression of a desire to die that will outlast the attempt.

While particularly evocative, situations involving suicide may clarify many of the limitations of our current thinking when it comes to decisions about life support therapy. In the aftermath of attempted suicide, it's tempting to stop treatment rather than to acknowledge and see beyond the grief. A typical attempt at suicide, if taken as a binding opinion that life should end, represents an extreme version of inauthentic autonomy. While other decision-making circumstances are less stark than is the case after attempted suicide, the risk of fostering a superficial rather than robust authenticity is always present in the ICU.

While I dive into the history, significance, and limitations of advance directives in the next three chapters, here I want to be clear about a central point. Many generous people with the best possible motives have advocated living wills and related documents for the last forty years. They are intelligent, compassionate people who are working toward worthy goals. Their work on advance directives has helped move culture forward in several important respects, even if the directives themselves do not work well. Despite these good intentions, the advance directive system itself is largely ineffective and in some instances dangerous.

Advance directives have created a moral hazard. Such moral hazards often arise when excellent aspirations and simple solutions run up against a more complicated reality, and they can worsen when culture changes. There was a time when living wills contributed meaningfully to important conversations within American society. There was a lot to digest culturally in the 1970s and 1980s. While many problems remain in our culture, living wills appear to have outlived their usefulness.

My argument about the experience of life-threatening illness and our need for new solutions unfolds in a series of chapters that move toward a vision for the future. In chapter 1, I describe the history of our approaches to death within American culture, with a special focus on the changes that occurred in the early twentieth century and the rise of modern ICUs. In chapter 2, I tell the history of advance directives, including the problems they hoped to solve and the goals and assumptions that shaped them. In chapter 3, I discuss the empirical and ethical problems that make living wills generally ineffective. In chapter 4, I explore the aspects of human cognition and emotion that also limit the usefulness of living wills. In chapter 5, I describe the experience of life in the ICU and talk about the ways that the ICU stacks the deck against the careful thinking that could preserve autonomy. In chapter 6, I explore the nature of life after life-threatening illness. I also discuss several of the recent innovations in the care of patients and families after an ICU admission. In chapter 7, I survey the current state of attempts to improve medical care for life-threatening illness and the culture in which it occurs. Finally, in chapter 8, I describe several new directions we should consider as a society and as a medical system. In an epilogue I share some practical advice about how to approach the possibility of life-threatening illness.

Three notes on terminology are in order.

First, I use the word "family" to refer to the people who matter to the individual patient. Many writers have tried to get around the association of "family" with the Victorian nuclear model: mom, dad, and several children, all living in a house with a white picket fence. In my research and reform work, I have participated in discussions about how to communicate respect for relationships that don't fit the Victorian mold. "Care partners," "loved ones," "friends and family," "informal caregivers," "members of intimate social networks" have all seemed serviceable to someone at some time. Yet nothing has worked quite as well as the term "family." "Family" has a complex history starting with large Roman households, which included all of the individuals attached to that household, regardless of the specific nature of their relationships. In one attempt to explore this question, colleagues and I settled on the phrase "the individuals whom the patient would want involved in his/her medical care."[5] I think that phrase captures what matters most, but it takes a lot of words to say it. So when I say "family," that's what I mean.

Second, because living wills and other advance directives share so much in common and because "advance directives" may sound technical while "living will" is familiar, I sometimes use the term "living will" as a shorthand for other advance directives. Where important differences exist, I employ more precise language to distinguish among the various advance directives available.

Third, in one of many absurd failures of euphemism in medicine, many physicians have come to call the decision to allow a natural death "withdrawal of care." To resist this tragic infelicity, I use "treatment" or "therapy" where usual sources might refer to "care" or "medical care." When we come to allow nature to take its course, we must be absolutely clear that all of us, clinicians and families, will continue to care for the person who is now dying. Even when we stop traditional medical treatments, we must always care.

Finally, a note of warning. I argue that living wills fundamentally misunderstand who we are as people: how we think, what we hope for, what matters in our lives. This misunderstanding contains several important risks. I worry most about the ways that this system subtly influences our behavior in ways that hurt everyone involved. The moral hazard encourages clinicians to cast patients and families adrift, guideless, in a muddled sea of tragic choices. Clinicians may learn from living wills that their uncomfortable duty to walk with patients through the valley of shadows is discharged by a signature on a legal document. Instead of sharing the confrontation with life-threatening illness with patients, instead of guiding people through a traumatic situation in a way that respects their autonomy and individuality, the system encourages medical professionals to tick controversial treatments off a checklist and walk away.

There is a place for something like advance directives as part of life's final wrapping up scenes for individuals with terminal illness, especially as part of an integrated system of delivering "palliative" care, treatments intended to improve comfort near the end of life. Individuals with terminal illness need and deserve devoted guides long before they might reach the ICU. When they are well supported, people very late in life will often reject what the ICU has to offer. Where such decisions honor patients' individuality and autonomy, they should be strongly supported. But living wills should be at most the trace or echo left by something much more substantial, a process of ongoing communication and guidance that begins early in the course of any life-threatening illness, whether it comes quickly or slowly.

Because I know it best, because it is the location in which living wills are generally meant to apply, and because the fundamental problems are so clearly expressed there, I use the ICU as a way to think more broadly about the ways medical professionals can be present with patients during serious illness. Some people will find that their life is near its end. The medical system must be responsive to their requests in ways that respect their individuality and ease their passing when the time comes. The strict distinction between living and dying that has been drawn so often in discussions of serious illness is not tenable. Living and dying are profoundly interconnected, and they often overlap. Both call for community and authenticity; both call for individualized guidance when health is threatened. Both call for honesty and introspection rather than talking at cross-purposes.

By means of this book, I hope to participate in the shaping of a new generation of health professionals attuned to the human needs of people navigating a life-threatening health crisis and newly empowered patients and families better able to persuade the system to serve them well. I am advocating reform that means something. Part of making these changes is bringing health professionals and laypeople to common understandings. As we acknowledge the shared humanity of physicians and patients, we make possible a human ICU. I intend to provide a common understanding for clinicians, patients, and families. I do not assume that readers will have any special medical knowledge; in footnotes I point to the relevant scientific literature for those with an interest in the technical side of things. Reading together will, I hope, be a prelude to walking together through the valley of shadows with our humanity intact.

PAST

Chapter 1

A Culture in Crisis

"Dr. Brown, we're sort of having a crisis. We found Mom's living will, and it says 'no life support,' but we've already been at this for ten days." Anxiety flooded Beth's face as she stopped me in the hallway outside bed 9 in the Shock Trauma Intensive Care Unit where I work. A thirty-something finance professional, Beth looked as if she were confessing a terrible secret.

Beth's mother, Martha, was mostly comatose. She had severe pneumonia, and our machines had temporarily taken over for most of her organs. Although I was not her primary physician, Martha's family had graciously enrolled her in one of our research studies, and I was touching base with them regarding the study. I reassured Beth that typical living wills rarely apply to patients in modern intensive care units (ICUs), but that I would review her mother's documents carefully to be sure her wishes were respected. Her features lightened visibly.

It didn't take long to read Martha's living will, which was typical of the advance directives I see in my practice. At a literal level, it was a stock legal form with her initials next to "My health care provider should withhold or withdraw life-sustaining care" followed by the signatures of two witnesses. Looking beyond the legal language, though, Martha's living will contained a plea to (1) not be maintained as a "vegetable" and (2) not have the dying process needlessly prolonged. As I discussed the document with Beth and her brother, they confessed that they had found their mother's living will a few days prior but hadn't found another physician in the ICU with whom they felt comfortable discussing it. I was flattered and horrified at the same time, glad to be of help but worried that our ICU had failed to meet their needs for communication and support at a time of great stress. They should not have had to wait several days to talk with someone about how to proceed with their mother's care in a way that honored her specific values, goals, and priorities.

Their discovery of the living will, itself not directly relevant to her current medical treatment because none of its criteria were met, gave us an opportunity to talk honestly about the chance that Martha might die. As recently as the 1980s Martha would probably not have survived even in the best ICU. But with advances in medical technology, today as many as eight out of ten such patients ultimately recover, even if they spend a catastrophic month or more on life support. Martha's children, however, in the absence of *any* discussion with her medical team about the possibility of death, were left to assume that she was certain to die. Beth and her brother were miserable at the thought that they were cruelly prolonging their mother's death. Their pain was very real, and the medical team's failure to communicate made it worse.

Martha's children were not overly pessimistic; typical of many families, they filled the medical team's silence with worst-case scenarios. They assumed their mother was dying but couldn't be sure. They were afraid that their discovery of the living will would result promptly in their mother's death.

To everyone's great relief, Martha survived. But many people in her situation do not. And at the time of the conversation about the living will, we didn't know how Martha's ICU stay would end. Except in very rare circumstances, physicians are not able to say with certainty whether any given individual person will live or die. That fact does not give physicians permission to hide from important conversations during life-threatening illness. It would, I think, be reasonable to describe this problem as a crisis, as the experiences of Martha and her children are repeated endlessly across America. Their stories are mirrored by dark stories of patients who undergo unchosen treatments that distort and deform their dying process.

It was just this drama of painful decision making when life is threatened that motivated the development of advance directives. To understand where advance directives have failed and what we could do to replace them, we have to understand where they came from and why. I acknowledge again here that many kind and thoughtful people have supported advance directives over the years. Whatever replaces advance directives will need to come to terms with their original goals—enhance patient autonomy while limiting paternalism, avoid the deformation of death through overuse of medical technology, and give people some sense of control over their lives—because those goals are worthy and important.

I begin with just enough history to make sense of the rise of advance directives. Living wills and the other advance directives that followed them reflect a specific cultural and historical context. Arising in the late 1960s with slow evolution through the following four decades, living wills represent an attempted solution to specific problems in twentieth-century American life. Three key elements played a significant role in creating the context in which livings wills aimed to transform society: the Dying of Death at the beginning of the twentieth century, the rise of ICUs and their associated life support technologies, and the dramatic social upheavals of the 1960s.

HISTORICAL DEATH CULTURE AND THE DYING OF DEATH

Throughout most of human history, societies have invested considerable cultural resources in making sense of our mortality. Societies and the cultures that support them approach the problem in many different ways: rituals, texts, social organizations, and holidays, to name a few. The rituals to manage the reality of death vary, sometimes dramatically, but almost every human society has had something like a script that helped people make sense of dying and death.

Some death rituals appear quite odd to Westerners—the rum-enhanced orgies and cattle wrestling that mark the funerary rituals of the Bara people of Madagascar are among the most striking—while others are more familiar.[1] The Bara drink copious quantities of rum to allow their ritual to unfold and to enter alternate states of consciousness. In this state, many have indiscriminate sex to affirm that life will go on, that death does not ultimately conquer humanity. They also wrestle cattle as an expression of human strength and will in the face of physical extinction. As strange as Bara funeral rites seem, these are rituals that affirm life and acknowledge the fracture in society introduced by each death. Western funeral rites have generally tended to be less physically strenuous than the Bara, but the fundamental concerns are quite similar.

By the time European colonists had established outposts and then their own country in North America, Western culture had settled into an approach that historians call the "good death." The idea behind the good death was that the deathbed was a time of moral and spiritual clarity. The dying had special wisdom to impart, and friends and family had obligations to the dying. Coming to terms with your own death and wrapping up your spiritual affairs were high priorities. To die in your sleep without forewarning (medieval culture called this the *mors repentina*, the much-feared "sudden death") was considered a curse because it stole from you the opportunity to complete your life's course and make peace with God. The good death was at once intensely religious and melodramatic. Loud, persistent mourning was encouraged, even expected.[2]

In the late nineteenth and early twentieth centuries, Western culture changed dramatically in several important ways. Death at an early age became less common, Progressive reformers believed they could fix most or all of society's ills, public health improved sanitation and introduced vaccination, and physicians finally began to have something to offer people, with an associated improvement in their reputation and prestige.[3] These and related social forces led to what historians call the Dying of Death, a sea change in society that separates us culturally from our predecessors.

The Dying of Death is of more than academic interest: We cannot understand where we are if we do not first understand how we got here. The historian James Farrell has done the best job of telling this story.[4] The process of eliminating death from polite society, by his account, stretched from around 1880 through the beginning of the Great Depression. That period in our history has become such a cultural wall that is difficult for us to see past it. Our culture is so different from the cultures that came before ours in that crucial respect that we often fail to understand what our ancestors' words meant. No matter how near America's "founders" seem to us in some current political discussions, the world they inhabited and many of their ideas and beliefs were not ours, not by a long shot.

The older culture of the good death was never about wanting to die, a point that many historians have completely misunderstood. Even in the good death culture that came before, people were not eager to die. The good deathbed was never suicidal. But when people came to die, they were able to create meaning. They were able to play their part in the drama centered at their passage from life to death.

Before the Dying of Death, death was a part of everyday experience. Death was recognized as horrifying, but people were able to understand it as part of the overall meaning of life and knew how to prepare for it when the time came. The understanding of death was broad enough to cross religious boundaries. The good deathbed was nondenominational, even if groups argued occasionally about which church did a better job of preparing its members for their ultimate confrontation with death. People certainly mourned, but mourning had a clear place in society. Those who mourned knew how to do it, and those around them understood what to do to help the bereaved. The good death culture included special status for the bereaved, a clear understanding of the needs of mourners, and a large community of those who had experienced bereavement. Before the Dying of Death, there were special mourning departments at the major department stores which stocked all the paraphernalia: dresses, veils, arm bands, black-rimmed underpants, rings, gloves, and necklaces that marked both the fact and the phase of bereavement. Even total strangers knew that a man with an armband or a woman with a black dress merited special treatment and consideration because they were bereaved.[5]

By the end of the Dying of Death, Americans had contained the terror of death by simply ignoring it until the moment of crisis, but the sanctity of death had disappeared along with its menacing presence. People found themselves newly unprepared when they came to die. Where many generations of humans had spent most of their lives preparing for their deathbed, modern Americans spent only hours to at most days, right in the midst of their death agony, trying to come to terms with what was once called the King of Terrors (a name drawn from the Bible's Book of Job). Since twentieth-century Americans had not generally spent their lives in the shadow of death, when they came to approach death, as every human being inevitably does, they discovered just how culturally defenseless they were before its terrible power.

So, how did we arrive at the culture that we inhabit today? Therein lies a web of interesting stories.

As reformers of various stripes, both religious and secular, began to improve living conditions and overall health, people rightly saw those innovations in a positive light. Hospitals became more common, and they had more to offer patients. Public health projects meant fewer people died prematurely. With time, safe and clean surgery raised the prospects of cure for several once-fatal conditions. We as a nation began to live longer, to die young less frequently. Scholars call this change in mortality the demographic transition, the point at which most deaths stop being associated with infection, trauma, and childbirth and come instead to be associated with cancer, heart disease, and strokes.[6] Although physicians made the occasional contribution, by and large the decrease in premature death came as a result of public health efforts: a safe food supply, clean water, reliable sewage processing, effective vaccinations, and improved roads and infrastructure.[7] The median lifespan jumped from around forty to about sixty years, with further dramatic increases soon to follow.[8] Diseases that still afflict the residents of many poor countries today, such as cholera, malaria, and tuberculosis, became bad memories in North America.

At the same time that life expectancy improved, the care of the dead became more professional. During the Civil War, undertakers made possible the movement of soldiers' bodies from Southern battlefields to Northern graveyards, and after the 1860s these professionals had more and more to offer the general public. The parlors in private homes, soon renamed "living rooms," ceased to function as places to pay respects to the dead. Instead, the dead were taken to freestanding "funeral parlors." Death became more professional, less domestic, less familiar.

Over the course of the Dying of Death, as the historian Emily Abel has made clear, hospitals became large and established institutions. Hospitals had historically been designated for indigent care, but they increasingly accrued power and authority as institutions that provided specialized care to patients from all sectors of society. Hospitals achieved sufficient size and ubiquity that they were forced to take over care of the dying. They didn't actually want the business; increasing social pressure prevented them from discharging the dying to other institutions, try as they might.[9] For some decades that is how it remained. Americans tended to die alone in a hospital bed, separated from family and home, often in great pain. The dying—once celebrated as people with special wisdom who deserved the rapt attention of family and even strangers—had become America's dirty secret. Skeletons in the nation's closet, and they weren't even dead yet.

Critics of our modern death culture have sometimes looked to the past as if a simple return to the prior culture will solve all of our problems. It has become a kind of squishy dogma that if we could restore the good death, medicine would be cheaper and people happier. They would not be inclined to pursue expensive, painful life support therapies near the end of life if the good death returned. Peace and happiness would be restored. But people have deeply misunderstood this foreign culture from the past. In the age of the good death, people would not have refused risky life support therapy. They would have embraced it. Good dying was never about refusing medical care. People who could afford it almost always hired a physician in the hopes of averting death. The medical care at the time was not terribly effective, but occasionally people sometimes recovered from life-threatening illness anyway. Good dying was based on a belief in Providence, the possibility that death could have meaning because it was part of a divine plan. Good dying provided a method for allowing human agency to become irrelevant and to trust in what God had in store. This Providential reasoning meant that there was a way for people to ultimately come to terms with death when all options had been exhausted.

Trusting that death could finally make sense allowed people to come to terms with dying, even to prize the process of coming to terms with it. Such trust is now rare. A major problem in contemporary society is that we combine our distaste for struggle or pain or disability with an unspeakable fear of death. This deep confusion can prevent us from wrapping up our lives and makes it difficult for us to find a healthful way through any life-threatening illnesses that we may survive, albeit with disability.

This denial of death and loss of expertise about the end of life are not the only reason that living wills seemed necessary. These cultural changes were important, but there were many other moving parts in the machine that became American society and its medical establishment in the second half of the twentieth century.

LIFE SUPPORT AND THE MIRACLES OF RESUSCITATION

Stories about reanimation are old. Gilgamesh in ancient Babylon, the prophet Elijah and the widow's son in the Hebrew Bible, Jesus and Lazarus in the Christian Bible, all highlight the persistent importance of stories about individuals brought back from the dead. In our contemporary world, those ancient stories seem rather unlikely, although in fiction, resuscitation is alive and well. We seem to live in an age of zombies and vampires and other visitors from beyond the grave. There is no image quite as striking as a person risen from the dead.

We tend to feel queasy about people brought back from the dead: Until recently zombies and vampires were not teen heart-throbs, but dangerous, malevolent beings. In most human cultures, people spanning the boundary between the living and the dead were some of the most frightening creatures known. Such individuals suggest that death may not be permanent, that there may be avenues of contact between the seen and the unseen worlds. There's nothing quite like seeing the dead rise to change one's opinion of the possible. But historically resuscitation has mostly been fodder for miracle stories, myths, or ancient traditions. Resuscitation from death has not been what typical human experience is based on.

This was true until the twentieth century, when a couple of technologies were perfected to the point of allowing something like resuscitation to occur. To some observers it might as well have been voodoo.

There are, of course, many reports of medical resuscitations over the long arc of human history. No one is really sure what to think of the older reanimations. Looking back from our contemporary vantage point, many of these accounts reported in older sources were probably related to temporary coma or perhaps a low heart rate that resolved on its own. (Before electronic pacemakers, it wasn't so strange for people with failing electrical wiring in the heart to have episodes of coma or near-coma that got better on their own after a few frightful hours.)

The oddest stories are the tales, probably mostly legend but not strictly impossible, of people found lacing their shoes during their own wake. These bizarre stories of reanimation almost certainly represent problems with diagnosing death—modern data suggests that one traditional method, feeling for a pulse in the wrist, may miss the time of death by days because blood pressure too low to feel at the wrist can still maintain the circulation[10]—and such diagnostic problems led to the occasional misperception that someone who had died had returned to life. (The availability of copious alcohol at wakes may have facilitated some of the remarkable reports, although that is pure speculation on my part.)

Over the short term, states halfway between life and death do exist. The brainstem has a response that researchers call "autoresuscitative breathing," in which the unconscious body takes deep, panting gasps, and that gasping can be enough to restart a heart under certain circumstances.[11] I have seen the occasional young person with very severe brain injury spend several hours in a condition that would have been diagnosed as death a century ago. Each time the person appeared to die, the panting resumed, followed by recovery of the pulse.

When I talk about resuscitation, I'm not talking about mistaken diagnoses of death. Today, we diagnose death more accurately than a century ago, but every once in a while even today a physician or other medical professional misdiagnoses death, albeit usually by a few hours at most. The final stages of the function of the heart and lung can sometimes still confuse even trained professionals. These misdiagnoses are not what I have in mind.

As physicians came to understand the body's final moments better, they diagnosed death more confidently, but they also began to discover ways to intervene in the process of death to interrupt that once-inexorable process. Starting with bizarre and ineffective methods like flogging the skin or hanging the patient upside down from his feet, physicians acquired options for responding to apparent death with techniques to restart hearts and take over for lungs that were temporarily not working. Over time these therapies and a system to support them coalesced into ICUs. This long history came to a kind of fruition in the 1960s and 1970s. We are now living out the ramifications of those decades.

THE RISE OF INTENSIVE CARE
AND "LIFE SUPPORT"

We would be wrong to think that our separation from death and dying merely arose as a result of advances in medical technology. The dramatic changes of the Dying of Death were already complete by the time physicians actually began to have useful treatments to offer their patients. In fact, physicians (as opposed to public health workers) only really began to have effective treatments after World War II, when developments related to the war effort and the rise of industrial science in America helped further medical progress. Physicians were still as likely to maim you as help you in the 1920s. While occasional advances, like surgery for appendicitis in the 1880s or insulin in the 1920s, did begin to help, by and large physicians had little to offer before 1960.

For most of human history what we think of as "doctors" weren't terribly distinct from magicians or snake oil salesmen. In the early 1860s, Harvard medical professor Oliver Wendell Holmes commented that if the drugs prescribed by his physician peers were sunk to the bottom of the sea, "it would be all the better for mankind, and all the worse for the fishes."[12] He wasn't much of a doctor himself, and he was prone to bouts of hyperbolic criticism of his fellow physicians, but in this instance he was essentially correct and would be for decades to come. Although his colleagues shouted him down, angry that he had accused them of dangerous incompetence, it wasn't until the middle to late twentieth century that his criticism no longer applied. Not to put too fine a point on it, but physicians were mostly bad for your health until the recent past. The Baby Boomers are really the first generation born under the aegis of modern medicine.

A combination of antibiotics, better surgical techniques and attention to sterile surgery, public health campaigns, and aggressive social campaigning led to the social dominance of American doctors. While physicians acquired prestige and social authority long before they made actual contributions to health (some argue that we physicians still mostly ride the coattails of public health, although that's not entirely fair), eventually physicians did have something special to offer. Open-heart surgeries, antibiotics for pneumonia and other infections, and chemotherapy for certain types of cancer all gave people new leases on life. Heart transplants especially captured the American imagination, even if they didn't work well in the beginning.[13] With time, medicine expanded to have something useful to offer even in the throes of acute life-threatening illness. The new technologies clustered together in ICUs.

Originally, ICUs were established for three types of care: surgical, cardiac, and respiratory.[14] First among those were postsurgical monitoring units, such as for patients with wartime trauma or recovering from large surgeries, beginning in the 1930s. One particularly horrifying fire outside Boston led to the existence of an impromptu burn unit at Massachusetts General Hospital for two brutal weeks in 1942.[15] Many scholars suggest that outlines of such units were visible in Florence Nightingale's attempts, during the Crimean War in the 1850s, to keep her sickest patients closest to the nurses' station so that they could receive prompt care when the need arose. These antecedents over time evolved into the surgical ICUs of the present day, in which nurses and doctors support patients through the turbulent aftermath of major surgeries.

Roughly in parallel with the evolution of surgical ICUs, a handful of cardiologists began to understand how to keep a person alive for a few minutes after the heart had stopped—and then, crucially, how to resume the heart's normal beating. This collection of techniques, now called "cardiopulmonary resuscitation" (CPR), has a fascinating history. Cardiopulmonary resuscitation and dramatic applications of electricity soon led to the second kind of early ICU, the cardiac ICU. The idea behind the cardiac ICU was similar to the surgical ICU: a way for medical professionals to watch closely for the development of an emergency.

Initially, CPR was almost exclusively for show. In its very earliest phases, one strain of CPR involved blowing tobacco smoke into the patient's rectum (for now-forgotten scientific reasons, it made sense at the time). By the early twentieth century, doctors were no longer blowing smoke up patients' tailpipes but were now cutting open the chest and squeezing the exposed heart by hand (in limited circumstances this is still done today; it's a staggeringly strange experience to squeeze another person's heart in your own hand). Eventually physicians figured out how to circulate blood by rhythmically pushing on the intact chest, what they called "closed chest" massage, as opposed to the prior open chest technique, in which physicians had cut between the ribs in order to place their hands directly onto the heart. These measures were just ways to buy time; on their own they did not restore life.[16] Restoring a nonbeating heart to life would in general require the highly coordinated use of electricity.

It took centuries to move from early observations about electricity's relationship to muscles to the successful application of electricity to a person's intact chest as a way to restart a nonbeating heart. In the nineteenth century, people observed that the limbs of dead animals could be made to move by electricity. By the early to middle twentieth century the use of electricity made plenty of scientific sense when it came to rebooting a short-circuited heart.

Through the 1930s researchers electrically restarted hearts in animal experiments, and slowly they began to apply electricity directly to the exposed human heart. The practice at the time was the rough equivalent of cutting open the chest and firing a TASER into the heart. The brutality of the requirement for opening the chest and touching the heart directly made this technique impractical in most circumstances. The Cleveland surgeon Claude Beck began publishing failed experiments with restarting a heart with this approach in 1936, but it was not until 1947 that he could finally report having saved a life with the technique. After a child's heart stopped during surgery to remove his breastbone, Beck spent almost an hour squeezing the heart by hand before he provided life-saving shocks, apparently related to delays in gathering the necessary equipment.[17] In 1960, after some early work in 1956, Paul Zoll and his colleagues in Boston demonstrated the viability of a technique for providing electric shocks across an "unopened" chest (similar to the advance in cardiac massage), reporting on a total of twelve patients in whom the technique was "successful," although only a couple of those patients actually survived the experience.[18]

"Defibrillation" became increasingly standard through the 1960s, delivering an apparent miracle to patients otherwise doomed to die. Then and now, defibrillation is a time-limited, emergency therapy. There were ever only a few minutes in which this electrical procedure could have a meaningful effect, before the lack of oxygen-rich blood delivered to the brain became fatal.

The development of successful electrical treatments for the arrested heart and the short time window in which it could be performed became the impetus for development of "coronary care units." At first there were no reliable therapies for heart attacks other than treating the associated rhythm disturbances with electrical shocks, so the main reason to develop a coronary care unit was to provide easy access to specially trained nurses who could immediately provide the shocks. People who were once consigned to immediate death seemed to rise from the dead. Patients who had by all traditional accounts died, however temporarily, were now laughing and eating and walking about the hospital wards. That striking image has entered our cultural consciousness as one of the most powerful medical miracles. The newly dead could rise again with CPR.

The third type of early ICU was the respiratory care unit, which was originally designed to support people whose respiratory muscles were paralyzed by poliomyelitis. Although it had been clear since the physicians Paracelsus and Vesalius in the sixteenth century[19] that bellows inserted into the windpipe could support an otherwise breathless animal, it was not until the twentieth century that the mechanical ventilator became useful and safe in human beings. (Some adventurous folk had experimented with bellows placed into other orifices, including the anus, based more on enthusiasm than wisdom.[20])

Blockages of the upper airway, as happened in severe cases of diphtheria, led to creative efforts to place a breathing tube through the front of the neck directly into the windpipe. First attempted in the sixteenth century, the procedure became much more commonplace in the nineteenth century. This "tracheostomy" was a tricky and dangerous technique, but when it worked it was lifesaving.

Surgery—once a wild ride with a bottle of whisky, a leather strap between the teeth, and a surgeon in a great hurry—improved dramatically after the 1846 introduction of ether, a gas that induced temporary unconsciousness. Over the next century, surgeons and now anesthesiologists experimented with ways to get patients ever more deeply asleep without killing them. Slowly, it became both possible and desirable to place breathing tubes through the mouth into the windpipe and then hook those breathing tubes to basic ventilators. Patients could be placed in a temporary, breathless coma, while the mechanical ventilator kept them alive through surgery. Those surgical ventilators were difficult to use, often unreliable, and only applied in brief surgical operations, but they were a dramatic improvement nonetheless.

Poliomyelitis, a foodborne illness that once caused widespread paralysis, provided the crisis necessary to push new ventilator technologies beyond their limited areas of application. For years, polio paralysis had been treated with the "iron lung," a giant vacuum tube into which a patient was placed feet first, with just the head protruding, like a turtle's. Theoretically, the vacuum kept the lungs inflated, making it easier for a patient to breathe, although iron lungs didn't work terribly well in practice. Physicians in Europe and the United States had experimented with inserting breathing tubes into the windpipes of patients who were dying despite the use of an iron lung, but it was the Copenhagen polio epidemic of 1952–1953 that ultimately transformed the world of respiratory intensive care. During the Copenhagen epidemic, the infectious disease physicians usually responsible for polio care called on an anesthesiologist named Bjorn Ibsen to try to contain the effects of the disease that threatened to kill the large majority of their patients. Following the lead of a handful of other physicians, Dr. Ibsen attached patients to systems that blew pressurized air into patients' lungs. The system used "positive pressure," while the iron lungs used a vacuum outside the chest to draw "negative pressure" to keep the lungs open.

Because electric ventilators were still in primitive form and limited supply, Ibsen called on medical students, about 200 of them, to assist with the breathing for the polio patients. Twenty-four hours a day, the medical students squeezed bags attached to the breathing tubes to blow air into patients' lungs, while Ibsen measured the levels of carbon dioxide in patients' blood. Carbon dioxide is the exhaust gas from the body's metabolic furnace, and the lungs must exhale it regularly or it will be converted to carbonic acid and the blood acidity will increase dramatically. Carbon dioxide accumulates when the respiratory muscles are weak and dissipates when ventilation is sufficient. Too much ventilation, a common problem when overzealous medical students created the breaths with their bags, inadvertently decreased blood flow to the brain. Too little ventilation resulted in death from buildup of acid in the blood. Ibsen's group dramatically increased survival during the epidemic, launching the lung component of what most people mean when they talk about "life support" therapies.[21]

The mechanical ventilator solved one problem and presented another, as it made it possible to prevent or delay death long enough for nutrition to become an issue. The artificial feedings that any extended period on a ventilator required have their own parallel history. Dieticians sometimes point to the ancient use of nutritious enemas as evidence of the antiquity of the craft, but enemas represented a lot more than just "feeding" the patient. Even if we ignore the enema antecedents for artificial nutrition, it is clear that physicians were trying to feed people through tubes into the esophagus, stomach, or small intestine by the sixteenth century. By the late nineteenth century, as surgery was just starting to resemble modern practice, several options became viable for artificial nutrition.

These techniques were intended for young children who were malnourished or dehydrated, for individuals who could not swallow (such as those suffering from tetanus or diphtheria), for patients whose bowels were temporarily dormant after surgery, or for people with severe illness of the digestive system. One frightening treatment applied in prisons in the late nineteenth century was the reversal of a stomach pumping technique to force-feed patients who refused to eat in the psychiatric asylum. The reverse pumping, according to one doctor, was a "perilous" task that could asphyxiate patients: he reported one death from drowning by beef broth.[22] For listless children, "gavage," placing food directly into the stomach via a tube placed through a nostril, was reasonably well established by the early twentieth century. Once ventilators and life support had made life with impaired consciousness possible, the gavage techniques seemed natural and were quickly applied to ICU patients. Although the method was artificial, food and water seemed as natural as apple pie and a glass of milk. This image would figure disproportionately in the debates that ultimately drove advance directives.

By the 1960s the three basic types of ICUs were reasonably functional, and lives were actually being saved in them. With this dramatic power to save lives, doctors pushed the boundaries between life and death, creating states of physical existence that had never been possible before. And with that ability came some undesired side effects and moral crises, the ethical quandaries that led to advance directives. Knowing when physicians were needlessly treating a dying person and when they were saving a life had become very complicated.

One story goes that physicians were distant from society, drunk with the power of their new techniques, and difficult to control.[23] There is probably a kernel of truth in that claim; doctors sometimes did apply their techniques in ways that didn't improve health or honor dying. In a 1956 paper demonstrating that defibrillation could work without cutting open the chest, Dr. Paul Zoll reviewed the fates of four individual patients. Of the four, three were already clearly in the process of dying when Dr. Zoll and his partners shocked them repeatedly; only one had even a chance of survival even if Zoll's procedures were effective. In a 1960 follow-up report, they described another eight patients, one of whom received 300 shocks before dying four months later at home. Over the coming decades, countless people in the act of dying would find physicians temporarily interrupting that inevitable process.

One account has become an emblem of that period. A British physician complained in a pointed 1968 letter to the *British Medical Journal* about the barbarous treatment inflicted on a colleague in America who was dying of stomach cancer. Pleading to be left alone to die quietly, this physician with cancer nonetheless underwent a procedure to open his chest and then endured extended life support despite what appeared to be brain death. His treating physicians added several miserable weeks to the process of this unfortunate man's departure from life. The British physician and his readers stood aghast at the inhuman behavior of the ugly Americans. Yet the kind of interventions decried in that now famous letter, "Not Allowed to Die," would only increase over time.[24]

A couple of problems burned especially brightly, as Western society tried to make sense of the new life support technologies. Physicians wielded considerable power, and society ostracized the dying. Those two social conditions, coupled with concerns about the authority of religious traditions and worries over the price tag associated with the new technologies, created the world in which living wills came to make sense.

The authority of physicians had grown dramatically by the middle of the twentieth century. Physicians by the 1960s melded together the moral authority of a secular clergy with the technological prestige of medical science.[25] This combination proved difficult to resist. Under this philosophy of "paternalism" or "parentalism" (the gender-neutral term), the medical system saw patients as children, powerless to over-rule the dictates of a parent. Most physicians didn't mean to be crass. They saw themselves as providing a needed service to vulnerable indi-viduals at a time of crisis. But the power that they held was dramatic and, in retrospect, dehumanizing.

Simultaneously, physicians were, if anything, even queasier about death and dying than their patients, who were already in deep denial about it. For physicians, death was a sign of shameful professional failure. There could be no question: Whatever the cost and whatever the context, physicians rejected death strenuously. While there were certainly pockets of deep humanity within medicine, reading the lit-erature from the period one is left with the image of a sort of Island of Dr. Moreau. Mad scientists created new generations of monstrous beings, although in this case, what the physicians were creating was people in a prolonged and uncomfortable state halfway between living and dying.

In practice, most physicians resisted pointless medical treatments, though they did so on an ad hoc basis, generally in secret. Some hospi-tals notoriously used removable purple dots attached to charts or eras-able pencils or chalkboards as ways to communicate among healthcare workers without ever letting an outsider—crucially, patients and fami-lies were considered outsiders to their own care—know what decisions had been made.[26] Patients had no real say in their treatment. Often they weren't even told that they were dying, based on the widespread belief that bad news could harm a person and even, perhaps, become a self-fulfilling prophecy. Doctors thought they were doing a service for their patients and families by keeping them in the dark. They believed that they were nourishing hope.

These problems were real and serious, calling out for change. Reform would require, as it so often does, a change in the cultural context for the problem.

LIFE IN THE 1960S

Among the many disruptions of the 1960s, the advent of the modern ICU might not immediately seem momentous. People remember the decade for America's rise to global power, the Cold War, and the mounting disaster in Vietnam. The nation experienced second-wave feminism and the struggle for civil rights. It was the rise of the so-called Pax Americana, in which American military, scientific, and industrial power established a new world order, albeit one clouded by a simmering hostility and nuclear arms race with the Soviet Union. The culture wars began to take shape, as the new left and the new right carved out their territory[27] and began to contend loudly about sex, abortion, and euthanasia among other issues.

The advent of the modern ICU was in some respects just as significant—it represented medical science's potential to maintain biological life beyond any prior barriers and necessitated a new definition of death. A half-century after the Dying of Death, this shift came at a time when Americans found themselves more and more skeptical about the moral trustworthiness of their physicians, who behaved like a new aristocratic class at increasing distance from the rest of society.[28]

This brave new world of medical denial of death was not without its critics. In 1955, the social anthropologist Geoffrey Gorer published an essay called "The Pornography of Death." Gorer had watched his sister-in-law dissolve into a nervous breakdown after her husband died. In mid-twentieth-century England, no one knew what to do with this grieving widow, least of all Gorer's sister-in-law herself. There were no social cues to guide their responses to her. Her world had been disrupted horribly by the loss of her husband, but in place of useful support, neighbors and coworkers offered only uncomfortable and isolating silence. Driven by the tragedy of his sister-in-law's self-destroying grief, Gorer set to thinking more carefully about the nature of dying in modern Britain. Something felt deeply wrong for him about a society so afraid of death that it abandoned its widows.

Gorer was a convinced Freudian and liked to apply psychoanalytic techniques to anthropological problems. His essay on the "pornography" of death uses psychoanalytic jargon that is now heavily dated, but his fundamental insight was spot on. In the Victorian era, you couldn't even mention in polite company that you needed to void your bladder or suggest that you knew that people wear underpants. But you could talk endlessly about death and corpses and death rattles and mourning practices and canes made from coffin woods or art made from dead people's hair. In the modern West, however, the situation had reversed completely. You could talk constantly about sex with impunity. You could use sex to sell products as banal as laundry detergent. But if you mentioned a word about death, people would stare at you as if you were a lunatic. Gorer's insights got people thinking broadly about cultural change and how to resist the stigmatization of death.

Gorer and others initiated a modest reform movement within Western culture. Some authors used fancy terms like "thanatology," or "death awareness"; others called it old-fashioned common sense. Whatever name they used to describe their apparently new but actually quite old way of talking about death, each of these people defied the legacy of the Dying of Death.[29]

The Swiss-born psychiatrist Elisabeth Kübler-Ross took a particular interest in death and dying, and in her now-famous *On Death and Dying* she laid out her "Five Stages" of coming to terms with death. When Kübler-Ross arrived at the University of Chicago in the 1960s, she found a medical establishment wholly unable to confront death or the dying. Organ systems and maladies had replaced human beings in Western biomedicine; clinicians and researchers pursued treatments for all the diseases that caused death rather than acknowledge that we were all ultimately mortal. The dying represented a medical failure that needed to be pushed from sight and memory. Medical schools paid almost no attention to the care of the dying. While Kübler-Ross later moved into some fringe philosophies, her activism on behalf of the dying mattered a great deal. The language she used to describe the process of coming to terms with death made dying people visible again. Her work directly promoted the spread of the hospice movement in the United States.

Across the Atlantic, the nun-turned-nurse-turned-physician, Cicely Saunders (made a Dame by Queen Elizabeth II in 1979), created the modern hospice movement to provide compassionate, effective care to people nearing death.[30] Kübler-Ross and Saunders amplified each other's work in a loose collaboration across the continents. Back in America, Jessica Mitford led a famous assault on the funeral industry, the professional group that had assumed control of the dead from family members. While she had very little useful insight about the process of dying itself, Mitford focused attention on several abuses committed by the funeral industry.[31] What she did not seem to fully appreciate was the extent to which the funeral industry was merely following the lead of the broader culture. While they threw a healthy dollop of philistine consumerism into the mix, funeral directors were mostly meeting America's cultural demand to not be exposed to death directly.

As critics of government and religious power joined with those who urged more soulful treatment of the dying, the question of how one dies and whether death could be chosen began to burn more brightly. Soon a variety of legal mechanisms arose to try to take power back from physicians and reassert human considerations when death is near.

Chapter 2

The Rise of the Living Will

In August 1967, Alice Waskin, not yet sixty, lay dying of leukemia in Wesley Memorial Hospital in Chicago. Suffering from intractable pain and with her physicians apparently reporting that she had just days to live, she attempted to end her life with an overdose of sedatives. Before hospice care was widely available, the dying often suffered feelings of agony and acute powerlessness, much like those Alice reported to her family. For some, suicide seemed the only possible escape from pain. Alice's attempt to cut short her suffering failed, though, and she recovered from the overdose only to plead with her husband and son to end her life by some other means.

Unable to bear his mother's pleading for death, twenty-three-year-old Robert brought a 22-caliber pistol to her hospital room. He kissed his mother goodbye and then shot her three times in the head, behind the screen that separated her from three other beds in the intensive care unit (ICU). Walking out of the ward, Robert laid the gun down and said "she's out of her misery now." He was arrested immediately, and a grand jury delivered a rapid indictment for murder. The case dragged on, as court cases often do, for a couple years, even though Robert never denied killing his mother.

By the time the case came to trial in early 1969, Robert's defense team had concluded that they would plead temporary insanity. While it seems unlikely that anyone believed the insanity defense to be literally true, the narrative was a persuasive one: His mournful sympathy for his mother overwhelmed his natural resistance to murder. Driven mad by the intolerable tension of his mother's deathbed suffering, Robert was not accountable for her homicide. In less than an hour, the jury set him free, having fully accepted his defense attorney's account of the situation.

The Waskins' story opened an influential 1969 law article that in some respects launched the advance directives movement. In it, Luis Kutner, a famous human rights activist and cofounder of Amnesty International, laid out a proposal for what he called "living wills." Kutner's personal story informs the story of the documents that followed and the culture that would come to support them.

Luis Kutner grew up in Chicago in the early twentieth century, graduating from the University of Chicago just before the Depression at the age of nineteen (he reportedly started college at age thirteen). He made his way as a defender of the individual against governments, at times tilting gloriously at windmills in the spirit of Don Quixote, but often making dramatic improvements in people's lives. Although Kutner never won the Nobel Peace Prize, he was nominated on multiple occasions, in celebration of his inspiring fight against oppressive governments. A detail that stands in for so much else in Kutner's life is his service as Ezra Pound's defense attorney, helping to free the famous poet from the psychiatric hospital where an embarrassed US government held him, pretending he was insane so that they wouldn't have to execute him for treason. (In a disturbing but all-too-common combination of narcissism and myopia, Pound had propagandized for Italian fascism during World War II.)

In his work at Amnesty International, Kutner repeatedly took on governments that were abusing individual citizens. His life's work bore a recurrent theme: protect the individual from powerful bureaucracies. "Speak truth to power," as the saying goes. Over time, he began to see medical treatment of the dying as a similar problem, one in which powerful physicians and hospitals were providing expensive and painful treatments to individuals who didn't need or even really want them.

In his 1969 law article introducing living wills, Kutner reflected on his own experience with a friend's slow and painful death, while also invoking recent prominent mercy killings, the Waskins' case being first among them. Kutner saw the living will as a "declaration for bodily autonomy" to protect people from unwanted violations of their privacy when they were unconscious. He saw such protections as "due process of euthanasia," by which he included both active euthanasia—mercy killings—and passive euthanasia—allowing an individual to die through refusal of life-prolonging treatments.

Kutner did not himself create the text of a living will, he just proposed the legal concept. Euthanasia activists were the first to implement Kutner's vision. They saw it as a compromise solution that fell short of the active euthanasia they had been advocating for decades but still a lever to move culture toward a broader embrace of death. The earliest living wills to gain much traction came from the Euthanasia Educational Council. A 1973 Dear Abby column strongly endorsed a "Good Death" (euthanasia) as a "human right" in response to a letter from "Concerned in Miami." Abby thereby created a bully pulpit for the Euthanasia Educational Council's living will, which declared that if "there is no reasonable expectation of my recovery from physical or mental disability, I request that I be allowed to die" and requested medications to "alleviate suffering" even if that treatment might "hasten the moment of death."[1] While that specific living will was soon replaced by documents that less explicitly stigmatized disability, a complex relationship between advance directives and disability persists to this day.

Occasionally, echoes from the Dear Abby column are heard today. I recently treated Roberta, a ninety-seven-year-old woman who was bleeding to death from a torn vein in her colon. She'd been in the hospital for two weeks for moderate kidney failure and was then transferred to a nursing home. She was back a day later, bleeding profusely. Her four children, all in their sixties and seventies, were terribly weary as I introduced myself to them in the ICU waiting room. I described Roberta's current situation and likely plans for her treatment.

Her family looked like they had something uncomfortable to say. I gave them space to wonder out loud whether death might be near, and they immediately reported that Roberta would welcome a natural death. "She even has this living will thing that she carries in her wallet," her son told me, withdrawing an item from his pocket. It was like a time capsule. Typewritten with an actual typewriter, on a crisply scissored half of a notecard, was the text of the Euthanasia Council will as published by Dear Abby.

Roberta's children already knew her mind, and the living will didn't technically apply to her situation because she was not unconscious or permanently disabled. But something important was missing from her treatment: No one had identified a crux moment, what I call a "clinical crossroads." Because she wasn't receiving life support per se, for two weeks no health professional had mentioned the possibility of allowing a natural death. Even while I was treating her, she was not receiving life support treatments, just blood transfusions and a colonoscopy to stop the bleeding. The living will had almost certainly come up in conversations—she was even DNR/DNI ("Do Not Resuscitate"/"Do Not Intubate"). But nobody had looked under the hood of those legal documents to understand what was deeply meaningful to Roberta and her family and how she currently understood her phase of life. After careful discussion with her family and me, Roberta chose to die naturally, without further medical interventions, and she enrolled in a hospice program.

Roberta's experience came decades after Kutner introduced the living will. Even as it pointed out some limitations of those living wills, the fact that Roberta had held onto that piece of paper for many years suggested some of the emotional power of such documents.

At least as it applies to allowing a natural death, Luis Kutner's actions moved a kind of legal reality forward. As living wills began to circulate and culture continued to change, several legal precedents established the basis for a legal doctrine of living wills. Yet, while the court cases are the usual starting point for discussions about the history of advance directives, nonlegal culture probably matters more. The court cases don't make sense except as reflections of and contributions to broader social and cultural currents.

After the Dying of Death, the dying had been separated from their families, robbing them of the resources necessary to preserve their dignity and comfort. Physicians had become socially powerful, and the hospitals in which they practiced had, begrudgingly, become primarily responsible for the dying. Physicians had developed the capacity to cheat death biologically, for many years in the lucky few, but only for a brief period in most patients. Those apparent medical victories often carried the cost of significant pain, suffering, and expense for the dying and their families. Simultaneously, dramatic social changes, including a push toward a more secular view of life and death and the rising distrust of the power of physicians, strengthened a desire to protect individuals from forces beyond their control.

THE FINDINGS OF THE COURT

While we tend to remember prominent court cases as if they were major drivers of social change, court decisions more often follow the broader culture. Judges are as much products of their society as anyone else is. It wasn't until the civil rights movement and the associated social change that courts began to acknowledge their prior failures to protect minority rights. It took the suffrage movement to persuade the courts to endorse voting rights for women. In general, a society—or at least an influential segment of society—develops its sensibilities to the point that a court decision can follow its lead. Still, court decisions do have a way of both distilling the opinion of our best legal minds and creating the authority of precedent. When the dominoes have been set up, a single falling piece can drop several hundred others. In the case of living wills, the effects of legal decisions were often incremental or primarily symbolic, but those court cases have provided a kind of language for discussing advance directives.

A handful of dramatic court cases centered on attractive young people who had lost all higher brain function after devastating accidents or illness. As these patients and others like them demonstrated, a person's status after the loss of human consciousness seemed to be at the whim of faceless medical and legal systems. Living wills promised to give individuals some hope of control over their own fate in the event of such a disaster, but at first they were not very widely accessible and considerable uncertainty persisted about how to interpret and use them.

The widely reported and closely followed experiences of Karen Ann Quinlan and Nancy Cruzan shaped our early understanding of advance directives.

Quinlan, a vivacious twenty-one-year-old, passed out after a party in the spring of 1975. Sedatives she had taken recreationally stopped her breathing, and she suffered a cardiac arrest from which she never awoke. She was permanently unconscious, and in 1976 her family received permission from the New Jersey Supreme Court to let her die by taking her off the ventilator. In an emotionally devastating reminder of how difficult it is to foretell the future, Quinlan spent another nine years in a nursing home, off the ventilator but still unconscious, before finally dying in 1985.

Tube feeds kept Quinlan alive those nine years after the ventilator was removed and became a major point of contest in the debates over medical interventions. The mechanical ventilator was obviously artificial, but what could be more natural than food and water? (The fact that tube feeds taste like sour glue hasn't distracted from that basic point.) Was the tube feeding of certain ICU patients simple and necessary care for vulnerable individuals, or was it cruelly and artificially prolonging the body's dissolution through artificial medical treatments?[2]

Nancy Cruzan, a twenty-five-year-old Missouri woman, was in a permanent vegetative state after a car accident in 1983, but she had no long-term need for a ventilator. Courts in Missouri refused her parents' request to let her die because she didn't have a living will. The US Supreme Court in 1990 issued a 5:4 decision that sided with Missouri's requirement that "clear and convincing evidence" be provided before allowing natural death to occur but simultaneously provided momentum for the notion that refusing life-sustaining treatments—even tube feedings—was both legal and appropriate. In Cruzan's case, apparently, all that was missing was a piece of paper.

Once the Supreme Court ruled, however, the judge in Missouri found a way to circumvent the need for a document to provide the necessary evidence. He accepted retrospective reports of conversations with Nancy Cruzan regarding her disinterest in life without consciousness that he felt were close enough to the "clear and convincing" standard. He therefore allowed Cruzan's family to stop tube feedings and she died twelve days later amid "pro-life" protests similar in fervency to antiabortion actions.[3]

The cases of Quinlan and Cruzan appear in almost every bioethics textbook and review article about refusals of life-sustaining medical treatments. These young women and their slow, painful-to-watch departures from life are justly famous. They galvanized attention in part because they were young, attractive people who were first normal and then profoundly abnormal.

The debates over the fates of these women relied on two different ways of seeing them: were they disabled individuals needing protection or dying people being tortured? There was a fine line between the two. As with most fine lines, the debates were less about the specific matter at hand and more about the cultural sensibilities and sensitivities that people brought to the argument. The general need to support disabled individuals was always clear, but people entirely bereft of consciousness didn't quite seem like the typical person with disability. They seemed more like dying people. Nevertheless, some observers thought that stopping feeds for Cruzan was tantamount to starving a disabled child. Many laypeople found arguments about the loss of personhood for unconscious individuals (a standard philosophical explanation for why people in permanent vegetative state weren't like other disabled individuals) an evasion, even as most felt that it was okay to allow someone to die if she was left in a permanent coma. The framing profoundly affected responses on this question. It feels very different to refuse to feed a hungry person who cannot feed herself than to refuse to instill otherwise inedible nutrient slurries into the stomach of a permanently unconscious individual whose personhood is gone. The tension between these influential framings, combined with broader cultural conflicts, made it difficult to solve the problems posed by Cruzan's plight in a general way.

Life context mattered too in decisions about artificial feeding: The same act of infusing nutrition through a tube could be seen as feeding a helpless baby or torturing a dying individual, depending on the context. Life narrative was central to that context: It was seen as very different to have started life with profound cognitive disability than it was to have lived normally before becoming disabled.[4] Cruzan, for example, seemed very different from the children with Down syndrome that were once left to die. (Unethical by our current understandings, it was routine to allow newborns with Down syndrome to die well into the 1960s.)

The court cases agreed on a few essential points. First, the right to privacy includes the right to protect the integrity of one's own body; second, there is a general right of self-determination, and third, killing people is distinct from letting them die. Each of these points became central to the final consensus that—with or without advance directives—people have the legal right to refuse unwanted medical treatments. Furthermore, to honor the refusal of those unwanted medical treatments is *not*, by legal and social consensus, the same as killing the person. While many bioethicists have rejected the consensus about a distinction between killing and letting die (generally as part of debates about assisted suicide), it has seemed to work for most of the country.[5]

Given the general right to refuse treatment, the problem was whether and how incapacitated individuals could exercise that right. People in permanent vegetative state, the most extreme form of incapacity short of brain death, became the natural focus for such discussions. What medical procedures should be done to people in permanent vegetative state, and who had the authority to decide? No one wanted anonymous bureaucrats in control of their fate. But when the individual patient couldn't speak for herself, who would do the deciding? How do you honor self-determination when the individual in front of you is entirely unconscious?

Originally, a "best interest" standard applied for deciding on behalf of an unconscious patient. Knowing nothing about the individual's specific beliefs, values, and priorities, what would most people want done to them? Such had been the general practice in American medicine for decades if not centuries: The definition of best interest put long-standing practice into legal terms. In retrospect, "best" was always in the eye of the beholder, and in practice the doctors did the deciding. The best interest standard therefore reeked of paternalism to most nonphysicians. Something new was required, some approach that was more specific to a given individual and didn't involve handing the reins to the doctors.

Rather than asking what most people would want in a given circumstance, the "substituted judgment" standard suggested that surrogates and clinicians ought to try to discover what the patient would choose in the circumstance. Substituted judgment represented in essence a thought experiment: Imagine what the patient would want if she could rise, clearheaded, from the sickbed to comment on her current plight. Substituted judgment remained at risk for misinterpretation by physicians and family members: The thought experiment was harder to perform in practice than in theory. The failures of substituted judgment made the quest for another standard more urgent. Enter the concept of "precedent" autonomy.[6]

Precedent autonomy maintained that the individual could (and indeed should) make certain crucial decisions in advance, when in possession of her full faculties, so that her judgment could be followed in the event that she was no longer able to decide for herself. Those who proposed such standards hoped that precedent autonomy would be the ultimate trump card. Such expressions of autonomy before the event were the theoretical foundation for advance directives. The hope was that in place of a thought experiment, families and clinicians could read a document completed in advance to settle the troubling questions of how to proceed in the treatment of unconscious patients. Hopes for precedent autonomy soon met with the reality that opinions about hypothetical events generated well in advance generally didn't answer the relevant questions at the time actual decisions had to be made.

Precedent autonomy ended up taking its place as one of the methods by which substituted judgment could be guessed at, with the growing acknowledgment that interpretation was still required. For many critics of paternalism, leaving things open to interpretation created too much leeway for clinicians. In an attempt to prevent physicians from dominating the interpretation of precedent autonomy, advance directives evolved to secure specific authority for family members.

Despite occasional misgivings about the capacities of families to represent unconscious patients, advance directives increasingly focused on designating a "proxy" or substitute decision maker to represent the individual patient's interests and life philosophy. Legal statutes began to create specific mechanisms for identifying such individuals and assuring their rights to decide on behalf of the patient. Often using the "power of attorney" mechanism known from financial and estate transactions, such laws, whether combined with traditional living wills or not, made legally explicit the importance of giving voice to an individual through the members of her intimate social networks.

While it was impossible to know, rigorously, what an individual would wish for in any particular situation, some form of substituted judgment has long seemed to be the best option for framing the responsibilities of such a proxy or surrogate.[7]

Evidence quickly accumulated, though, that surrogates poorly understand patients' wishes and that they bear substantial psychological scars when they feel responsible for the decisions being made.[8] Wherever possible, proxies hope to avoid having to make those decisions and tend to mistake their own views for the views of the patients.[9] Many surrogates came away from the experience with diagnosable post-traumatic stress disorder.[10] On the other hand, some observers worried that families might be forcing physicians to provide aggressive treatments the patient would not want, and that proxy documents might introduce too much latitude.[11] Despite difficulties and misgivings, identifying a proxy was a nod in the right direction. The identification and development of a community for each individual is essential. Everyone should know who will accompany them in the valley of shadows.

There would be a lot more work to do to get the system to work smoothly, but a legal structure was established in the 1970s and 1980s that would last for decades.

LEGISLATION

To understand the legislative details of the advance directive movement of the 1970s and 1980s, we need to understand the social environment of the time. There was a move toward a stronger focus on the individual, and as culture increasingly championed the underdog, physicians were perceived as less trustworthy than they once had seemed. People also worried about the rising costs of healthcare. And the culture wars were underway, casting discussions about the "end of life" alongside debates over abortion.

As is often the case, the states paved the way for federal legislation. California started the trend in 1975 with the "Natural Death Act,"[12] a hybrid that was seen by its authors as giving physicians a way out of the "cul-de-sac" of technology that otherwise led to a medically disfigured death. The California living will, improving some on the Euthanasia Council precedent, established a stock form containing simple language to allow physicians to stop treatment of an unconscious individual.

Within just a few years, essentially all states developed their own legislation to support living wills.

Fifteen years later, shortly after Nancy Cruzan's death, Congress passed the Patient Self-Determination Act (PSDA) of 1990–1991, which attempted to put the living wills that had become commonly available state by state on a secure footing nationally. The PSDA required hospitals to develop written policies regarding advance directives; to advise patients, at the time of admission, that they have the right to refuse medical care through advance directives; to offer them such an opportunity; and to keep records of those advance directives on file. An unfunded mandate to educate the public about advance directives accompanied the legislation.

In practice, hospitals provided highly simplified versions of advance directives that designated a patient's "code status." "Code" referred to a hospital's system of emergency alerts—one of which was for the cardiac arrest of a patient. "Code" has since become synonymous with attempted resuscitation when a patient is not breathing and/or has no heartbeat. "Full code" meant hospitals should make all attempts at resuscitation in the event of a cardiac arrest, while "DNR/DNI" meant they were to make no such attempts. The enactment of PSDA looked to be one situation where Congress passed legislation that the country wanted and needed. Proponents of advance directives saw it as a clear victory: Laws should require powerful businesses to advise vulnerable people of their rights to resist exploitation. While, in retrospect, the PSDA didn't actually bring about much change, the legislation was symbolically very important.

These legal approaches to the question explain why many patients complete their living wills now as part of routine estate planning with their attorneys, with no relevant medical input or expertise. Bringing important questions about health into the purview of lawyers, legislators, and regulators has had some unanticipated negative effects.

DISCLOSURISM AND A FOCUS ON PROCEDURES

In response to unethical research and the pervasive medical paternalism of the first half of the twentieth century, America turned to what critics term "disclosurism" to regulate encounters between physicians and patients.[13] The important idea behind disclosurism is to provide the individual with all information necessary to an informed choice and then record the choice made. The devil, as so often, has proved to be in the details. Pursuit of disclosurism's good idea in society at large led to the End User License Agreements that we must pretend to read every time we purchase a computer program or log into a new web page. It's the philosophy that has brought us 100 pages of small type to sign when it's time to buy a house.

As Carl Schneider and others have commented, disclosurism saps people of autonomy at the same time it appears to be legislating that very autonomy. Drowning in unintelligible legal terms, people are left obligated by those very words they don't understand. The problem with disclosurism is that individuals are bound by the terms of contracts they can't possibly understand, but to which binding signatures are required. While most advance directives aren't quite as detailed as End User License Agreements or mortgage paperwork, they arise from the same legal thinking and have many of the same problems. The scientific evidence suggests that disclosurism does not bring the benefits people want from it, and does not protect their actual interests.[14]

As advance directives developed through the 1980s, they mainly increased their specificity in one way or another, adding ever more complicated disclosures or decision points. In 1989 Ezekiel and Linda Emanuel, both bioethicists and, at the time, a power couple in the field, developed what they called the "Medical Directive." It required individuals to scan through a range of possible medical scenarios based around imminent death or profound disability, and indicate which therapies they would accept under which conditions. Treatments and disease states are arranged as if on a morbid bingo board. Open spaces allowed the individual to select an option with an X. For example, C8 on the grid is "invasive diagnostic tests" for "brain damage" plus a "terminal illness" like cancer. Options that aren't even possible are blacked out, to keep patients from making impossible selections.

Like many societal proposals from physicians and bioethicists, the Medical Directive seemed like a sound idea in theory but was a dud in practice. The form was too complicated and inadvertently emphasized physician rather than patient perspectives. While the Emanuels allowed the option of a trial of certain treatments that would stop if they were not effective (in my experience, this is the option most people want), the Medical Directive blacked out that cell as an unavailable option for cardiopulmonary resuscitation (CPR). But for many patients, we don't know at the time CPR is performed whether it will result in satisfactory recovery or permanent loss of consciousness. Why not focus on desired outcomes and actual trade-offs rather than hypothetical refusals of particular procedures? While the Emanuels are intelligent, compassionate individuals who have made important contributions to medical ethics, their Medical Directive was not one of them.

Yet authors of other next-generation advance directives followed the Emanuels' lead, adjusting and revising at each iteration, sometimes for the better and sometimes for the worse. The end result in several living wills was a disclosurist tangle of options, which I've never actually seen used in practice.[15]

Most of the living wills still in circulation are little different from the originals, and the ideology is essentially unchanged. This reality contributed, inadvertently, to an important oversight of the Affordable Care Act (ACA). When President Barack Obama tried to incorporate advance care planning in the ACA, he personally completed a living will because it was "something that is sensible" to do.[16] This symbolic gesture was part of the support for a now-notorious early proposal within the ACA that encouraged physicians to have advance care planning discussions with their patients by offering a new billing code and imposing financial penalties for failing to obey the advance directives that resulted. Billing codes are the financial lifeblood of American medicine. The codes define what doctors get paid for, and doctors do what they're paid to do, just like everybody else. Accountability makes sense, too, at least in theory: We clinicians should be responsible for how well we do our jobs. The ACA's advance care planning proposal had two problems, though, one fixable, the other fundamental. The ACA proposed funding advance care planning discussions when most medical practices lacked the tools to do so in an authentic way. The lack of useful tools was fixable: Once you fund an activity with appropriate incentives, the tools will come. It's the American way.

The penalty ACA imposed for noncompliance, however, revealed a fundamental misunderstanding of the nature of advance directives. It's the relationship and conversation that matters, not the static, often uninterpretable stipulations of a legal form. Requiring clinicians to strictly obey the details of a directive drafted on the basis of speculative future scenarios would have made living wills actively dangerous rather than just distracting. Political partisanship obscured the fact that both the ACA and its critics were missing the point when it came to the duties health professionals owe their patients during life-threatening illness. The ACA was not proposing "death panels," but neither was its approach to advance care planning particularly wise in the current medical climate. The problems of making a flawed system even more powerful is a risk that has recurred as lawmakers have sought to improve the reach of living wills. (A somewhat improved approach to the problem arrived in late 2014, as Medicare directly proposed new billing codes to support advance care planning discussions with patients. The lack of truly useful tools to support these discussions remained a serious problem, but the billing codes are a step in the right direction.)

IMPROVING ENFORCEMENT

Shortly after they were introduced, it became apparent that advance directives were mostly toothless. The documents were often locked in a file cabinet at home or in a primary care office, unavailable to physicians in the hospital. In addition, because advance directives were instructions to a physician, they lacked the medical or legal authority to be implemented by nonphysicians. This mattered especially in a skilled nursing facility (medical professionals often call them SNFs, pronounced "sniffs," defeating the purpose of the abbreviation that replaced the already euphemistic term "nursing home"), where physicians were only occasionally present. A crisis in a nursing facility at night therefore meant transfer back to a hospital, because no doctor could determine whether the advance directive applied.

Problems with advance directives in nursing homes led to the development in Oregon of the Physician Orders Regarding Life-Sustaining

Treatment (POLST) paradigm, which basically made advance directives binding.[17] The POLST gave real teeth to advance directives: If you became sick at a nursing facility and had a POLST refusing hospitalization, the nurses wouldn't even call 911. The POLST represents a binding medical order rather than just instructions to a doctor. Those who thought that the main problem with advance directives was that healthcare professionals failed to comply with them saw POLST as a viable solution. Those who worried that advance directives poorly represent the preferences of the patients who completed them saw POLST as a real risk. Despite some skepticism, versions of POLST have become available in many states. This more aggressive stance on enforcement points toward the ongoing tension between individuals and society that permeates discussions about advance directives.

FUTILITY, FINANCIAL DISASTER, AND OBLIGATIONS TO SOCIETY

Over the last fifty years, difficult conversations about the obligations we all owe to society have run alongside conversations about an individual's right to determine what treatments physicians should provide. A communitarian ethic has always existed in parallel with the strongly individualist arguments in favor of living wills. A tension between community and individual perspectives is almost always present with advance directives. As the costs of healthcare have increased, certain treatments aimed at prolonging life in difficult circumstances came to be seen as wasteful. Why provide expensive ICU treatments for a patient whose cancer will soon kill him or a patient with advanced Alzheimer disease, especially if the person had doubts about whether to do them in any case? Advance directives came to be a way for individuals to vote for a national policy regarding limited medical resources. Through living wills, people could refuse such wasteful treatment in advance.

Whether the competing communal and individual currents within living wills represent incoherence or nuance depends on your perspective. But this ongoing tension contributes to the occasional, inflammatory association of advance directives with "death panels." While that rhetoric is not helpful, it is also true that when advance directives are violated it is overwhelmingly in favor of providing less rather than more treatment.[18] This problem of balancing the individual versus the community will always be present, necessitating honesty and transparency for discussions to be productive.

When the communalist approach to advance directives is invoked, the decision about treatment often turns on the question of "futility." The medical community strongly supported the focus on futility when it arose in tandem with living wills. By classifying certain treatments as futile, physicians reasserted their authority, because they were the ones who could decide whether certain procedures were thereby permitted. While the concept was dressed up in different ways, "futility" generally meant less than 1–10 percent predicted chance (the definitions varied) of recovery to life without disability. Where many patients saw a fight for life, physicians and ethicists saw wasted resources that we as a society could ill afford.[19]

Strictly speaking, a therapy is futile if it could never achieve its stated end. Administering Diet Coke in someone's veins to treat a heart attack is obviously futile. As is giving a person with pneumonia two pounds of blue cheese. There is no biological reason to think that those treatments would succeed: They are futile. Any success with such treatments would be best classified as a miracle or a hoax.

In practice, though, futility was almost always used to describe medical treatment about which physicians were pessimistic or that was associated with a quality of life that physicians thought was poor. These assessments of futility were prone to serious problems. Most importantly, they reflected the perspectives of clinicians rather than patients. They generally ignored the reality that many patients and families differed markedly from physicians in their thresholds for deciding what odds of recovery were sufficient to support continued medical treatment.

Even at a technical level, life support was almost never actually futile. In truly futile circumstances the designation didn't make any difference because that's what futility means: An effort cannot make a difference. For those reasons the concept has faded from ethics, although in my experience many clinicians still use futility to express their uneasiness about care when the stakes are high.[20]

The research used to make arguments about the costs of futile treatments also suffer from a problem with their methods. Specifically, futility assessments were made in retrospect, on the basis of a death, regardless of the predicted survival at the time the decision to treat was made. But the actual decisions about whether to treat had to be made prospectively, on the basis of patients' goals and the likelihood of meeting those objectives. The decisions made at the time affected both those who ultimately died and those who would have died without treatment but didn't. While some authors criticized the research behind futility, it continued to play a role in discussions about advance directives.[21]

Methodological problems were compounded by the fact that futility is, in large part, a way to talk about rationing medical resources without having to address the controversial question head on. It allowed physicians to express their distress in ways that ran counter to the honest desires of patients and families. While any given patient only had to endure a single difficult illness for a modest probability of success—not remotely futile, from the patient's perspective—clinicians were haunted by the cases in which treatment did not succeed. Futility became a way to drown out patients' voices.

I talk more about clinicians' moral distress in a later chapter, but we have to candidly acknowledge the reality of what is often called "rationing." The idea behind rationing is that a limited resource has to be shared, and we don't always get everything we want. We ration healthcare already, largely based on whether a person has insurance, or when they show up for treatment, or how sick they are. "First come, first served," means that the patient who arrives at the hospital on a Tuesday after a busy Monday may not get one of the available ICU beds. It's already a fact of life.

There are ways to frame rationing that are more helpful and less helpful. "Death panels" is not helpful, but neither is the usual failure to acknowledge that a conversation is about rationing when in fact it is. Proponents of rationing—or of thinking more clearly about rationing— talk about our interdependence as citizens in a shared country, about the limited resources currently available, about the worthy efforts like vaccination or nutrition that go unfunded because we spend so much on Medicare for dying patients. These are important conversations to have, and they merit careful, honest communication, which is often not forthcoming.

However, even if cost savings makes intuitive sense, several studies suggest that advance directives per se have little prospect of saving money. Ezekiel Emanuel and others have demonstrated that the major expense near the end of life doesn't come in the ICU. They point to custodial care, mostly at home or in nursing homes as patients become progressively weaker, as the source of most of the expenditures in the last six months of life among Medicare recipients.[22] The reality is that as we become less independent with advancing age our care becomes more expensive, especially in our socially fragmented society. Even if we never use any life support technologies, it's expensive to house and feed and bathe us as we wrap up our lives.[23]

This is an important point, worth clarification. General concerns about limited resources and the expense of caring for older individuals near the end of life helps to drive the still ubiquitous idea that nursing homes are where people go to die. But Atul Gawande and others have argued persuasively that seeing life in a nursing home as intolerable often depends on debasing the value of the lives people lead in a nursing home.[24]

EXPANDING HORIZONS

Despite ongoing concerns about the expense of high-risk treatments and belief in the potential of advance directives, many observers soon recognized that more would be required than legal documents to meet patient's needs. Some of these individuals began efforts to change medical culture. Specifically, they advocated an approach to medical decision making that included more emphasis on patients' perspectives, while involving them directly in all matters that affect them. This movement toward "shared decision making" encompassed every aspect of healthcare, at all phases of life. In parallel with these developments, early work on hospice evolved into an entire medical specialty, "palliative medicine," focused on humanizing serious illness and easing burdens near the end of life.

Some associate the rise of shared decision making with the publication of the psychiatrist Jay Katz's influential *Silent World of Doctor and Patient* in 1984. Katz rejected physician paternalism in stark terms and argued strongly that in place of the traditional silence of the examination room, real, substantial conversations between patients and physicians were required. Researchers and activists responded to Katz's rallying cry and created a discipline to pursue rigorous approaches to decision making that balanced out the power of physicians. Rather than settling for disclosurism's legal forms, shared decision making tried to fine-tune doctor–patient interactions and be sure that patient voices were heard in real time.

Shared decision making was part of a more general attempt to put the patient at the center of medicine. As part of this effort, some institutions incorporated simple advance directives into a broader effort called "advance care planning." While the specific details varied from place to place, advance care planning tried to apply the principles of shared decision making to questions about preparations for the end of life. Some versions of advance care planning were little more than living wills plus a pamphlet or two, while others moved closer to a robust program of support through illness near the end of life.

The general philosophy underlying advance care planning overlaps some with a movement called "slow medicine," a health-focused variant of the "slow food" movement that preceded it. Slow medicine is a deliberate, patient-centered approach that doesn't rush to heedlessly perform procedures without reflecting on whether they are likely to realize people's goals.[25] What matters most in a slow approach to medicine is listening closely to patients and pausing before treating or testing to be sure it actually makes sense.

The goals of slow medicine were, in many respects, the original aspirations of advance directives. But the actual work of slowing down medicine demands much more from clinicians than handing out living wills. An entire infrastructure for support and care when life is near its end is necessary.

Prompt and attentive palliative care and/or hospice when the time comes are part of the labor required for a healthful, slow approach to both life and medicine. Hospice offers alternatives to a brutal death for people with terminal illness. It focuses on managing symptoms like pain or difficulty breathing, rejecting treatments that are no longer beneficial, and helping people find meaning in the final phase of their life. As hospice expanded, palliative medicine became the specialty for training hospice physicians as well as moving beyond hospice. While uptake has been somewhat tardy, important voices have supported the broad application of palliative care. In a recent, influential report, the Institute of Medicine advocated for both greater use of palliative care and an understanding that such care must encompass more than just medications for symptom control in the last week of life: People require social supports outside of clinics and hospitals to help them flourish in their own homes even when they are physically fragile.[26]

While the aspirations of hospice were laudable, the reality could be frustrating. The most common way to enter hospice was to be in the hospital, perhaps the ICU, when the doctors abruptly decided that you were dying and placed you in hospice for some morphine and Valium for a couple of days before you died. Some specialists and observers hoped that living wills could be a foot in the door when it came to conversations about the end of life, while others found them a simplistic distraction from more important work. Whether that was true or not, in hospice the problems were real and present rather than speculative and future.

Living wills were forged in the furnace of America's culture wars, in which conservative and liberal camps battled over abortion, euthanasia, disability rights, individualism, and the nature of community. These very public battles over morality and life and death revealed how often physicians had mistreated disabled individuals and research subjects. Americans decided that the law was the best way to restrain these medical professionals while it also sought to resolve social conflicts about the meanings of life and death.

Two groups of patients became the laboratory for this legal reform experiment: the permanently unconscious and the dying. Advance directives worked, sort of, in the case of the first, and this apparent success made it more likely that advance directives would be overextended in the second, where they didn't work.

Permanent vegetative state, first proposed as a syndrome by that name in 1972–even if it wasn't firmly diagnosable until a couple decades later—became the ideal test case for advance directives.[27] Karen

Quinlan and then Nancy Cruzan were both in permanent vegetative states; their cases focused the attention of the entire nation.

Patients in permanent vegetative state have no consciousness, just an eerie sleep-wake cycle and a collection of low-level reflexes that some-times mimic interaction. When cardiac arrest is the cause, essentially no one in a vegetative state for more than three months has ever awakened. When head trauma is the cause, it takes a full year to be confident that recovery is exceedingly unlikely.[28]

Return to consciousness from permanent vegetative state essen-tially never happens and in the rare circumstances when consciousness returns, there's very little of it. Still, the disconcerting sleep-wake cycle, the striking reflexes, and sometimes impatient physicians means that clinicians and families occasionally fight over what to do for patients in permanent vegetative states. Even though the large majority of vegeta-tive patients died peacefully and without commotion, rising distrust of physicians meant that the status of vegetative patients became a bone of social contention.

Several aspects of permanent vegetative state made it an attractive problem for advance directives to solve. Famous court cases addressed it, the syndrome was basically one thing that could be securely diag-nosed, there was some public legal controversy about what to do, and very few people ever wanted to be in it (public polls have consistently suggested that only around 10 percent of people indicate willingness to be maintained alive in a permanent vegetative state). In these con-ditions, advance directives proved reasonably useful, even though they were addressing an astonishingly rare circumstance.

Instead of the rare, clearly defined, and highly predictive situation of the permanent vegetative state, living wills were brought to bear in the ubiquitous human experience of death. While they apply in very rare circumstances, they are employed much more broadly.

Advance directives started with worthy aspirations and an admi-rable attention to the dignity of individuals. They were grappling with issues that rocked the nation, trying to answer questions about the meaning of life and the risks of medical technology. Simultaneously we as a nation were grappling with the relationships between individuals and their communities and the complex but increasing role of human agency in death. These were big problems, and they deserved careful attention. Advance directives hoped to be an answer to many of these questions. They probably did play a role in the early years in focusing attention on an important problem. High aspirations sometimes met with disappointing implementation. The promise of early legislation has now largely morphed into the almost farcical practice of physicians-in-training asking distractedly when patients are admitted to the hospital, "Do you want everything done?"

I admire the fervor of the early support for living wills. They represented a way for individuals to resist the tyranny of a dysfunctional medical system. Finally, there seemed to be an opportunity for a person's voice to be heard, an arrow piercing the armor of medical paternalism. Advance directives became the preferred mechanism to realize the ideals of autonomy and self-determination for patients. I believe that people ought to have their voices heard. I wholeheartedly support the goal of hearing people's voices and honoring their individuality at all times.

Because of their ubiquity and the current absence of viable alternatives, we as a society need to understand the problems with living wills in order to move beyond them. We need ways to live life richly and deeply in the presence of death and a medical system that can facilitate our flourishing. Because the ICU represents the technological battle with death and the setting for urgent difficult decisions about medical care, replacing living wills and repairing the ICU are dependent on each other. The goals were worthy even if the approach was heavily constrained by a given moment in American history. It really does seem true that substantial change in American medicine was overdue. Physicians were secretly making decisions about treatments and were widely separated from the rest of American society. The conspiracy of silence about death was very real. Physicians had in fact committed ethical abuses in research and experimental transplantation surgeries.

That specific cultural moment has passed. Living wills or no, it's difficult to conceive of a physician secretly refusing treatment anymore. The authority of physicians overall is much more limited than it was.

A key question to explore is whether advance directives represent a partial solution that ought to coexist with more sophisticated or integrated solutions. Or are they outdated techniques that can cause harm? If living wills only make sense in the presence of some other solution, that other solution can exist without living wills, and if the living wills cause problems when they are used in isolation, it may be time to retire them.

Unfortunately, evidence and experience suggest that living wills are the wrong tool for the task at hand—supporting people, specifically and personally, when their lives are threatened. Because so much of the medical and societal response to serious illness is based on these flawed, legalistic documents, I discuss their failings in the next two chapters.

Chapter 3

Empirical and Ethical Problems
with Living Wills

Fran, a third-year medical resident from Oregon, explained to me as I arrived to supervise care in the intensive care unit (ICU) for the night that her patient in room 506 was "DNI/chest compressions okay." She noted that fact with a scowl. "What a stupid code status," she explained, shaking her head in disbelief. "We can't intubate her, but if she arrests we can shock her and break her ribs and then leave her to die without an endotracheal tube? Stupid." Fran was right: The code status was stupid. But the stupidity belonged to the medical system, not to her patient. The system had set up both Fran and her patient, Belle Smith, to fail.

"Code status," a term of medical jargon, attempts to translate a web of human feelings and aspirations into a brief set of technical instructions for nurses and physicians. This fact is easily forgotten. Code status asks patients to make categorical decisions about highly specific medical procedures on the basis of hypothetical future health crises. Asking patients and families to do their own translation of their preferences into the technical terms of cardiopulmonary resuscitation (CPR) is unlikely to help people flourish.

Fran and I went together to speak with Belle. A woman in her mid-sixties, Belle had struggled a bit with her diabetes but had been mostly healthy before her current episode of pneumonia. She had claustrophobia and hated the thought of the breathing tube, which she remembered gagging her when she came out of anesthesia after gall bladder surgery. She said that waking up after surgery was "a total nightmare, choking to death on that tube and I couldn't say a word." As we explored her wishes a little more carefully, Belle made it clear that she also never wanted to end up in a permanent vegetative state, "like Terri Schiavo." (Schiavo, a young woman in Florida, suffered massive brain damage after cardiac arrest, and her husband and parents battled over her fate for years. Her case culminated in explosive legal and political debates carried out on national television.[1]) But, Belle said as we discussed her current medical situation, if she had a decent shot at recovery she would want aggressive medical care, including intubation and CPR with chest compressions. She just wanted help with her claustrophobia if it came to that.

We changed Belle's code status to "full," aware that if she reached a point where meaningful recovery was no longer likely, we would then transition to an exclusive focus on her comfort rather than continued life support treatments. We also promised Belle that we would use medications to keep her claustrophobia to a bare minimum if she did end up needing the ventilator. Fran moved from mystified to embarrassed to relieved as the conversation progressed. As best I could tell, it had never occurred to Fran that a "stupid" code status represented miscommunication rather than a willfully difficult patient. Honestly, I'd missed that same fact myself, often, over the years.

Fran, and the many other students and physicians I have worked with over the years, are good people who want to do the right thing. But they can be carried along by the inertia of advance directives. These young clinicians have become messengers carrying coded letters they do not understand. The messages are so wrapped in jargon and misperception that they remain hidden in plain sight. Well-intended healthcare workers tend to read code status instructions literally, without discovering the actual intentions beneath them; these failures make doctors and nurses complicit in a cruel system that paradoxically decreases autonomy. In most cases, code status and living wills end up providing uninterpretable answers to highly specific but rarely relevant questions. The process both muddles the conversation and leaves its participants believing a problem has been solved. "I'm glad we got that unpleasantness out of the way," everyone seems to think as they go their separate ways, without a clue about what just happened.

I think a lot about Fran and Belle. If Belle had suffered a brief crisis, the team might have let her die on the basis of a misleading code status. People want to avoid unnecessary brutality when their lives are threatened and to live and die in ways that are authentic to their values and priorities. Those are worthy goals that I wholeheartedly endorse. Unfortunately, for historical and technical reasons, advance directives tend to get in the way of those goals.

It has taken decades for people to appreciate just how poorly advance directives address the problems patients and their families actually face during life-threatening illness. As patients, families, and I make our way through the perilous waters of life-threatening illness in the ICU I am struck by the sad reality that, as a general rule, advance directive documents tend to substitute for and distract from careful thinking. Such substitutions are particularly risky for novices who lack the experience necessary to compensate for the failings of the documents, and most patients are novices when it comes to life-threatening illness.

More to the point, advance directives both reflect and reinforce a distorted view of how human beings make decisions and how they experience the stresses of life-threatening illness. Advance directives also generally fail to acknowledge the meaning of life lived in the presence of death. The reasons for these failings are many. Some are reasons inherent to living wills and the medical system, while others relate to how human beings process information. I focus on the structural problems in this chapter, and the human factors—mostly related to known limits to the ways human beings process information and make decisions—in the next. We start with a basic paradox at the center of living wills.

LIVING WILLS REPLACE PATERNALISM WITH A FALSE AUTONOMY

Disclosurism, the legal movement we met in the last chapter that employs legal forms to ostensibly empower consumers, creates a situation in which procedures intended to maximize autonomy may in fact imperil the very autonomy they aim to protect. The forms and documents and signatures and notaries of disclosurism are impressive, but they fail to answer important questions about human flourishing when life is threatened, and they often misrepresent the preferences they are trying to elicit.

I worry, quite a bit, about the difference between appearance and reality when it comes to autonomy. Disclosurism protects a nominal rather than a robust autonomy. In defense of a more robust autonomy, the Yale psychiatrist and law professor Jay Katz described "psychological autonomy" with an associated "duty to reflection," while the early English philosopher John Stuart Mill—a philosophical founder of modern liberalism—described the need for effort, expressed through meaningful conversations, to assure that autonomy is discovered and respected. In a compelling recent treatment, the psychiatrist Jodi Halpern described the need for clinical empathy to be able to assess honestly and accurately the meaning of a medical crisis with patients.[2]

These writers propose something very different from the devotion to the nominal autonomy that disclosurism advocates, but their vision has often been lost in contemporary medicine, in which two metaphors have dominated thinking about the relationship between physicians and patients. The old, paternalist metaphor that lasted into the 1960s was of the physician as uncommunicative parent, classically the father, unilaterally deciding what was best for the patient-child. The newer, consumerist metaphor is of physicians as producers and patients as consumers of goods, exchanging money for services in the healthcare market. Neither of these metaphors is satisfying. The better solution lies somewhere in the middle. I propose a different metaphor, that of clinicians as guides, as a way of acknowledging the robust autonomy proposed by Katz, Mill, and Halpern.

Mountaineering guides are well known for leading expeditions through potential danger to the conquest of high peaks. A skilled guide establishes goals with a client and then continuously interacts with him or her over the course of a climb. At times, the guide points out important risks to safety. In rare circumstances, to avoid a grievous, life-threatening error, the guide may even briefly overrule the client's inclinations. During an expedition, guide and client walk together, sharing a safety rope on the mountainside, and staying in communication. While the metaphor isn't perfect, it correctly emphasizes a working relationship that is based in mutual respect and constant communication.

Individualized, timely guidance is what we wanted when my wife was sick, and it's what most patients and families want in the ICU. When we were dealing with melanoma and the loss of Kate's eye, we didn't want a physician dictating to us what came next without any input, but we also didn't want what was offered instead, a couple of informed consent forms for surgery and an offhand comment about the possibility of molecular diagnostics. We wanted someone knowledgeable about the range of possible approaches to her disease who was willing to understand us as people and guide us in creating a map between our sensibilities and a given medical course of action. I believe strongly that such guidance would, in most cases, help to achieve a robust, deeply meaningful autonomy.[3]

The style of autonomy proposed by living wills differs strikingly from the autonomy supported by empathetic guidance. The specter of paternalism is partly to blame: Attempts at guidance could be exploited to tell an individual how to choose rather than helping her to choose a course of action that is true to her as a person. Fear of such paternalism has driven many ethicists to advocate a strictly procedural autonomy: If the forms are all in order, to put it crudely and a little unfairly, autonomy has been served.[4] But if the forms consistently mislead people, the flight from paternalism could threaten the goal of authentic self-determination.

While "authenticity" has become a loaded term, the fundamental idea behind authenticity is that something—a state of affairs, a decision, a way of presenting oneself to the world—is consistent with the actual, persistent beliefs and values of the individual.[5] Without wading too deeply into philosophical arguments, I see an authentic autonomy as an expression of one's will that is, to the extent possible, not swayed by framings or considerations that are alien to that individual.[6] This is what I mean by a robust rather than a superficial autonomy, and it's what I believe we should aspire toward as clinicians and others supporting individuals during health crisis.

Critics might see such a call for authentic autonomy as a kind of "soft" paternalism on a slippery slope toward hard paternalism. (In ethics, "soft" paternalism seeks to avoid deceit, coercion, or simple accidents that may threaten the integrity of an individual's self-determination; Mill famously used the example of preventing the use of an unsafe bridge when an individual walks toward it, not knowing that the bridge will likely collapse under his weight.)[7] Such a criticism would probably be misplaced. While I see a place for some "soft" paternalism in society, my concerns about living wills relate to the ways that they inadvertently imperil the self-determination they seek to support.

The disclosurist model of advance care planning incorporates considerations relevant to culture wars, legal norms, and physician biases in ways that ostensibly turn control over to the patient but generally do not. By offering inscrutable documents as if they are straightforward maps, living wills are the equivalent of turning the controls of an airplane over to a novice, with the auto-pilot silently turned off. The plane will crash, no matter where the person wanted to fly it. If these legal mechanisms—living wills—have effects on treatment decisions that give the appearance of protecting autonomy while actually undercutting it, then they are supporting an inauthentic rather than an authentic autonomy. Because disclosurism substitutes for and distracts from actual communication, it's extremely common in my experience that patients and clinicians believe that communication has happened when it never did. Because people assume that they are useful devices for communication but living wills only require a signature or two and checks in a couple boxes, they can lead us down a primrose path, away from authentic personalization and robust autonomy.

What will lead us back in the right direction is empathy, a key component of the kind of personalized guidance needed to preserve autonomy. Jodi Halpern frames her elegant and persuasive book on the need for such empathy in place of clinical detachment around the tragic case of "Ms. G," a woman who died from a thoughtless application of procedural autonomy. Ms. G's husband suddenly abandoned her after she lost her legs to complications of diabetes and kidney disease. The combination of spousal abandonment and double amputation left her emotionally devastated: She immediately became desperately depressed. She refused any further kidney dialysis, and her treating physicians resonated with her sadness, agreeing with her transient judgment that her plight was hopeless.

The autonomy paradigm told clinicians that if Ms. G said she didn't want dialysis, it wasn't their place to second-guess that proclamation; in Halpern's report, no clinicians engaged in substantial conversation with Ms. G. Yet by taking this approach, the medical team abandoned her, unconsciously siding with her husband and her own disempowering depression. Ms. G died shortly thereafter, as a direct result of stopping dialysis.

Halpern spent years pondering and mourning her role in the abandonment of Ms. G, and her meditations on this failure lead to a moving portrait of the need for vigorous empathy on the part of clinicians.[8] Halpern argues that empathy allows clinicians to help patients access an unfettered view of their own potential and their future. Although she wrote this before the "heuristics and biases" school of psychology (which I describe in the next chapter) had popularized new language to describe human thinking, Halpern was describing the importance of identifying certain irrationalities in order to support people in their attempts to make decisions that are consistent with their own values and priorities. In Ms. G's case, no one took the time to explore with her how she might learn to live again after her husband's betrayal. No one bothered to determine whether Ms. G's existential cry of despair was an authentic expression of her autonomy.

The nominal autonomy of disclosurism treats clouded acts like Ms. G's refusal of dialysis as if they were binding acts of self-determination. But an authentic approach takes the time to discover and review with the individual any threats to her autonomy in ways that support self-determination. No one even spoke with Ms. G for very long; they just backed away from her despairing sobs. The status quo approach often treats any document or stated preference as binding, no matter how vague, inscrutable, or misunderstood. Advance directives preserve the appearance of personalization and autonomy but not the substance. The better alternative is a deep and empathetic commitment to understanding the individual seeking guidance as she makes her way through the valley of shadows.

LEGAL DOCUMENTS MISS WHAT'S MOST IMPORTANT TO US

Empathic individual guidance is the gold standard for treatment, because legal documents like living wills so often miss the mark regarding the values that are most important to us. What's more, patients sense how artificial living wills are. They know how unlikely they are to address the nuances of a future medical condition. In one survey, many patients had no idea that the living will would apply in the circumstances where it was supposed to.[9] In other studies, only a modest minority of individuals who had living wills wished for them to be complied with strictly. Instead, they wanted their loved ones to make assessments at the time they actually need to be made; people don't generally want their hypothetical speculations to force a particular course of action in the distant future. For example, almost 80 percent of participants in one major study didn't want their directives followed: They hoped that physicians and family members would decide on their behalf instead. Another study a decade later of 337 people over the age of sixty-five found that fewer than 10 percent wanted their advance directives followed exactly. The majority of respondents wanted their proxy to have "a lot" or "complete" leeway for interpreting the advance directive.[10] These empirical data give the lie to claims that advance directives deserve priority over other forms of communication.[11]

As we've seen, living wills represent the fruits of the legal philosophy of disclosurism, and as a consequence they tend to obscure more than they illuminate. Relationships, sustained in real time, are much more likely to represent our aspirations than legal documents ever could. Such relationships, nourished by high-quality communication, are what matter most when it's time to wrap up our lives. But the advance directives paradigm insists instead on legal documents.

The foundation of this legalistic approach is a philosophical and legislative fiction. Proponents of advance directives have maintained that a legal document, however alien and prone to misinterpretation, must be more valid than conversations with friends and family. In one famous philosophical discussion, advance directives were considered a binding "performance," like a contract, rather than one piece of evidence about a person's opinions;[12] this precise claim stood at the heart of deliberations about whether Nancy Cruzan could be allowed to die in Missouri.

For some decisions—say, buying a house or a car—legal documents are in fact binding performances. Such contracts make sense when we are buying and selling things. "I will pay X dollars for object A or service B."

"We will publish this book or make this movie." Such contracts accurately reflect promises made about concrete present and future events. By analogy, living wills are often seen as contracts that state, "I forbid X, Y, and Z procedures be performed on future me in the event that I lose consciousness or am certainly dying." Such an analogy to contracts was a key component of the legalistic interpretation of living wills.

This central conceit, that a legal document is superior to human communication for relaying intimate values about health, has been repeatedly demonstrated to be incorrect. In fact people tend to pay much less attention to legal documents than to other mechanisms of communication.[13] The superstar geriatrician Joan Teno and her colleagues made this point clearly in a study of decision making among families of patients with serious illness. Study participants discounted the written instructions of living wills as generally irrelevant to decisions, in large part because the language of contracts does a poor job of communicating values and aspirations.[14] Indeed, the majority of living wills are comically unreadable legal documents. Several studies have confirmed what a cursory glance suggests: Only experts can understand typical advance directives. Living wills are documents written by lawyers for other lawyers. At a most basic level, the language itself is tough to fathom. The usual reading level of a living will is twelfth grade, while the reading level for most Americans is eighth grade.[15] Not only are the words themselves inaccessible, but their meaning in context also depends on expertise in both medical and legal jargon. After earning a bachelors in linguistics and spending a decade-and-a-half in medical practice and three years doing intense research on the topic, I finally feel competent to interpret a living will as a legal document.

Medical and legal cultures are far removed from the human values most relevant when life is threatened. By keeping the conversation focused on specific procedures rather than the life threatened and the individual's sensibilities about life, living wills paradoxically but predictably tilt discussions in favor of physicians. It's quicker and easier to talk about procedures than it is to puzzle together through the needs and possibilities of the seriously ill or to understand the rich mental and emotional life of an individual patient. With living wills, clinicians don't have to deal with the complex problems of actual communication—and this failure of communication can open the door for serious errors.

I've heard advance directives compared to seatbelts, a precautionary measure we employ in the rare event it will be needed. Most people don't crash a car, but some do, and seatbelts save lives in serious car crashes. The comparison is tempting. I'm sympathetic to that view: People do, very rarely, end up in a permanent vegetative state, and this is the situation that living wills might effectively address. But the comparison to seatbelts is misleading. In the event of actual crisis, living wills may malfunction seriously, causing harm. The more accurate analogy would be to seatbelts that inadvertently strangle the user during minor fender benders. They are a tool designed to help in rare circumstances, but they are capable of doing active harm. Alternatively, living wills represent a strange gamble: an insurance policy for an extremely rare event that penalizes you if more common events occur.

Living wills often fail to represent the values and priorities of the people completing them. The University of Maryland law professor Diane Hoffman asked 110 older individuals living in and around Baltimore to complete standard living wills at the same time they were interviewed about their wishes in the event of a medical catastrophe. Around half of study participants completed living wills that were at odds with their simultaneous stated wishes.[16] This finding confirms what other studies have shown: People often do not understand or agree with what they are signing when they consent to a living will. For example, a group of emergency medicine physician-researchers at Beth Israel Deaconess Medical Center in Boston found that "code status" orders commonly do not reflect patients' actual wishes. In 2011, they interviewed 100 patients newly admitted to the hospital with an existing Do Not Resuscitate/Do Not Intubate (DNR/DNI) order. They made sure that the patients were awake, not in physical distress, and able to think clearly. A researcher then described various scenarios to the patients to find out what they thought about being intubated or resuscitated under specific circumstances. They had expected that about 10 percent of patients would have a different view than their DNR/DNI order suggested; instead, they discovered that almost half of the patients they interviewed would want intubation, the precise opposite of what their DNR/DNI order said.[17]

The painful and sobering case of Hank Pinette should give all of us pause. An older but still independent Floridian, Pinette spent much of 2004 in the hospital for heart failure that wouldn't get better. He had signed a typical Florida living will in 1998 as part of routine estate planning with his lawyer. It stated that if there was "no medical probability of recovery" from a "terminal" illness, he did not want to prolong the process of dying. His physicians had come to feel that Hank's case was hopeless, while his wife Alice believed that she could still communicate with him and wanted to keep fighting.

Alice and the hospital reached an impasse and turned to the courts. The hospital's "risk manager"—a euphemism for the person whose main task is to limit a hospital's legal liability—petitioned the court to allow the hospital to stop treatment over Alice's objections. The judge agreed with the hospital ethics committee, composed entirely of hospital employees or medical professionals, and ordered the hospital to let Hank die.[18]

The Pinettes' case was one of the few circumstances in which a living will actually had teeth, and it gave a hospital bureaucracy power over Hank's emotionally traumatized family. If he'd been asked, Hank may well have said it was okay to continue treatment if his wife still had hope or would be upset if the hospital overruled her.[19]

Perhaps the most disturbing fact of the case is that it appears from available court records that no one discussed the matter with Hank while he was still awake and in the hospital. Instead of a direct, timely conversation grounded in what Hank could actually expect in his near future, the medical professionals relied on a six-year-old document he had completed without any input or assistance from trained medical professionals. If Hank was like most people, who don't want their advance directives strictly obeyed and certainly not over the objections of their designated decision maker, the court made the wrong ruling.

The stark black and white language of advance directives can cause other misinterpretations. Occasionally medical professionals are tempted to avoid useful therapy out of a fear that it might be burdensome, however temporarily. Jack, a dignified gentleman approaching eighty, came to my ICU after surgery to remove a diseased gallbladder. The anesthesiologist had removed the breathing tube as Jack began to awaken from anesthesia, but he was in the 1 percent or so who have trouble breathing shortly after the breathing tube is removed. This difficulty is almost always a temporary problem related to the lingering effects of anesthesia medications.

As Jack arrived in the ICU it was apparent that he was not fully awake or able to breathe on his own, but as I began to mobilize the resources necessary to reintubate him, a nervous resident informed me, with two medical students backing him up, that Jack was DNR/DNI and had a living will requesting no heroic measures. They felt that I should not reintubate Jack; they even seemed distressed that I would consider it. Over their objections, I reintubated Jack, who spent about a day on the ventilator. He went home four days later, in reasonable health, grateful for his brief stay in the ICU and the life it had allowed him to continue to share with his family.

Jack's case was a chance for my students to understand that they had seized on particular words or phrases torn from their original context, even as they tried to do their duty to the patient. Back when Jack completed a living will in which he tried to communicate that he did not want to live in a permanent vegetative state, he likely didn't imagine that his choices would influence a technical judgment about his care immediately after a routine surgery. Instead, he was trying to communicate that when it was his time to go, he didn't want the process artificially prolonged. These are very different things, but the legalism of the advance directive paradigm blurs the two. In Jack's case, healthcare workers very nearly honored a misleading "code status," possibly because his advanced age made it easier for the team to believe an ambiguous directive. As so many others, Jack's living will had created a situation he did not foresee, one that risked actively harming him. In the absence of an advance directive, no one would have objected to intubating Jack; it would have been routine.

These problems associated with misinterpretation are only intensified when advance directives must cross racial or cultural barriers.

The Problems for People of Color

The issues with living wills get more serious the further they get from the social context of their creators: wealthy white people. Overwhelmingly, advance directives have been tools for affluent, well-educated Caucasians. Many reasons likely contribute to these racial disparities— more comfort with the legal process, a greater sense of power and personal authority, and a belief that institutional power can be turned to their benefit rather than detriment. While such issues are complicated, it's probably true that differences in religion also play a role—affluent whites are generally less religious than people of color.[20] Some of the effect is probably also related to the difficulties of communication across cultural boundaries and knowledge about medical care.[21]

Whites are more likely than African Americans to stop medical treatment early after cardiac arrest[22] and are more likely to recommend against CPR when presented with a video simulation of a "code status" discussion.[23] Consistent with these observations, most studies suggest that African Americans and Hispanics/Latinos complete living wills at much lower rates than whites[24] for a variety of specific and culturally valid reasons.[25] In general, people of color don't want more legal forms—they often distrust the legal and medical establishments and for good reasons. As a rule, they want personalized, insightful guidance when their health is threatened.

Although education and wealth may well play a role, the noncompletion of living wills by people of color is more than an educational or socioeconomic issue. There is a profound philosophical difference at play here. In multiple studies and surveys, Hispanics/Latinos and African American much more often want all treatments to be applied when life is threatened.[26] In the 2013 Pew Research Center survey of attitudes about death and dying, four-fifths of whites agreed that there "are circumstances in which a patient should be allowed to die," while less than half of African Americans and only a third of Hispanics/Latinos agreed.[27] Most people of color disagree with the central requirement of the Patient Self-Determination Act (PSDA) according to one early survey: They don't even want to have advance directive discussions when they are hospitalized.[28]

Context matters, and people from different cultural backgrounds will have their own responses. Some early important work revealed that Mexican Americans believed that the doctors wouldn't offer something they didn't believe would work, Korean Americans wanted their families to speak on their behalf even when they were awake, and African Americans were extremely skeptical of the good intentions of physicians. The finding among Mexican Americans was particularly concerning, as it suggests that the standard approach to autonomy may lead to profound miscommunication: By neutrally listing off possible treatments to be accepted or refused, physicians may inadvertently endorse even treatments that they believe are very unlikely to work.[29]

Minority patients commonly worry in surveys that living wills could be used to deliver substandard medical care.[30] The fact that minority patients often receive lower quality care in general should worry all of us.[31] They have fewer options for a good death even when the decision has been made to allow a natural death.[32] In addition, the ethical breaches that led to living wills occurred in a culture that preyed heavily on minority communities. African Americans are often right to be skeptical, given the weight of history suggesting that American physicians have not cared well for African Americans.[33] A vast amount of work remains to be done to understand how best to support people of color during life-threatening illness. Standard living wills are not the solution.

In addition to the problems we've already seen with living wills not reflecting people's actual wishes and not accounting for the unique circumstances raised by racial and cultural diversity, living wills deal in hypothetical scenarios that rarely arise in real life.

PIG IRON UNDER WATER: THE CONDITIONS LIVING WILLS FORESEE ARE RARE

A focus on rare and dramatic cases, coupled with some basic cognitive biases, has left many people with the impression that living wills are likely to apply to them at some point in time. But that's just not true in the contemporary United States. For all the fear of permanent vegetative state, there are probably no more than 5,000 individuals newly diagnosed with permanent vegetative state each year, in a nation of 300 million people.[34] (Of those, almost half are children, who would not have completed an advance directive in any case.) Overall, that's an annual risk of about one one-thousandth of a percent. In any case, most people with permanent vegetative state will die peacefully without a living will, just as they did before Nancy Cruzan's case reached the Supreme Court. Almost no one is forced to persist in permanent vegetative state merely because they lack an advance directive. Insurance professionals call risks that low "pig iron under water," meaning they are as unlikely as submerged metal catching fire. Insurers would be more than happy to offer fire insurance on wet iron, but the insurance wouldn't be worth buying. Even Cruzan herself, after the Supreme Court upheld the stringent Missouri law preventing her death, was allowed to die without a living will.

The other specific situations envisaged by living wills are nearly as rare. The precise constraints that living wills impose on the dying process are almost never encountered in hospital practice. Dr. Joan Teno and her colleagues analyzed the living wills of participants of a large study of patients hospitalized with a serious illness. What they found was discouraging news for proponents of advance directives. The vast majority of directives said nothing that specifically applied to the patients' actual medical situations.[35] In 2011 a research group in Germany took another look at the problem that Teno first addressed in the 1990s. They asked how often living wills were or could have been applicable for patients admitted to their ICU. The answer was no more reassuring than Teno's: very rarely.[36] Most people in the modern West die without ever moving through a state of unconsciousness in the presence of healthcare workers in which their death is certainly imminent. They either die at home or on the highway, or their deaths are "negotiated" in the ICU before they ever reach a point of "certain" death, where "negotiated" is a researcher euphemism for limiting medical treatments in some way.[37]

There are too many different ways we become severely ill, too many distinct pathways through life-threatening illness, for advance directives to apply broadly. Even if we made living wills as detailed as the federal tax code, they still wouldn't cover most of the crises people face near the end of life because every situation is distinct.

Would we really want the equivalent of a tax form to be the way we confront our mortality as individuals and as a community? I doubt it.

The problem might be improved if patients and clinicians could accurately see the future, but there again, the data are disappointing.

PREDICTIONS ARE OFTEN WRONG

Because they are legal documents, most advance directives are designed to apply under very specific circumstances, much as business contracts, which stipulate: "When X happens, pay Y." "If I fail to provide A, then take B from me." In this respect, they are typical contracts. As opposed to other contracts, though, essentially all of the specific requirements of advance directives depend on predictions about the future. "Permanent vegetative state" is a prediction about the durability of a state of unconsciousness. "Terminal illness" is a prediction about near-term death.

But predictions are always inexact. The old saying reminds us, with a bit of a rummy wink, that "Prediction is hard, especially about the future." The art of prediction is just that: an art. Researchers have worked to make medical prediction more of a science, but they have made only minimal progress when it comes to the level of certainty that matters to most patients and families. Even top-of-the-line predictive modeling falls short of the certainty that would be required to make advance directives truly useful.

One morning in June 1978, William Knaus, a newly minted ICU physician, assumed care of a desperately ill young woman who was failing rapidly from shock after surgery to remove cancer from her ovaries. She died almost immediately thereafter. His physician colleagues hadn't noticed anything especially wrong with the patient overnight. As Knaus tells the story, this young woman's death only minutes after he met her shook him to the core. He realized, as he tried to process her sudden death, how little he and his colleagues could predict what would happen to any given patient.[38] Knaus set to work without delay applying statistics to the problem of predicting the future for ICU patients. The system he and his colleagues developed over the next several years— the Acute Physiology, Age, and Chronic Health Evaluation (APACHE) score—has evolved over several decades.[39] The APACHE II is still in use, but APACHE IV is available, and researchers at Oxford University are hammering out the details of APACHE V. Most US physicians who treat patients with life-threatening illness use or are familiar with some form of the APACHE system.

Predictive scores, like APACHE, and their acronyms reproduce rapidly, and dozens of researchers have proposed specialized versions for specific diseases. Belgian investigators proposed SOFA (Sequential Organ Failure Assessment), French researchers developed SAPS (Simplified Acute Physiology Score), and American physicians created the MPM (Mortality Probability Model). Those are only the best known of the general predictive models. In the area of pneumonia alone—what was once called the "old man's friend" because it was such a common way for older individuals to pass away—there are easily ten different models to predict mortality, with abbreviations as strange and diverse as SCAP, PSI, CURB-65, and SMART-COP.

While researchers often argue at length about the relative merits and demerits of the various models, for our purposes they are not all that different. All of the available models have been useful in some respects. Hospitals and ICUs use the models to compare the quality of the care they provide to the care provided at other hospitals nationwide. Without some kind of quantitative method for measuring how sick patients are, every hospital would blame their patients for observed death rates: "Of course we have more deaths; we're treating the sickest patients." Every hospital thinks its patients are the "sickest," so there has to be a referee of some sort, an external, quantified method to determine whose patients really are the most infirm.

The prediction scores do a decent job at this task because they tend, when averaged over large numbers of patients, to give accurate estimates. So if a hospital has a rate of death among its patients that is higher than what is predicted by the score, there is cause for concern. These prediction scores have other uses, all dependent on having large numbers of patients: health policy, resource planning, and scientific investigations of cause and effect.

Knaus and many others have hoped that the prediction scores could also help individual patients and physicians.[40] That is the holy grail of those scores. Providing appropriate and successful care for individual patients is what gets most physicians out of bed in the morning; their own specific outcome is clearly what patients value most, even if they are civic minded. But, for all the benefits of the prediction scores, that is the one thing they just can't do. Such scores and models describe large groups of people. Most careful statisticians have agreed that with rare exceptions, these scores are not useful for prognosticating a single individual's course with the certainty that matters to actual individuals needing to make decisions.[41]

Unless we understand something about the techniques used to build prediction scores, we will not be able to understand their limitations when applied to individuals. Fundamentally, the problem is that statistics is the science of large numbers, but every person is an individual, a "sample size" of one.

Most prediction scores use some version of a statistical technique called "regression." Regression methods define a straight line that best summarizes, in a simple equation, many measurements in a way that clarifies relationships among different elements or variables. The line is usually chosen to minimize how far the observed measurements (data points) are from the proposed line. In general regression "models" (a fancy name for equations) assume a basically linear relationship—that is, if one element increases, the other element increases by a proportional amount. In the real world, few relationships are actually linear, but the assumption works well enough for many problems.

Regression models are useful for discovering associations in large groups of people. Some of those associations are important (for example, obesity is associated with diabetes), while others are less so (death is associated with advanced age). But statistics is the science of large groups, not single individuals.[42] We don't know whether this man in the clinic will acquire diabetes because he is obese or that this woman in the hospital will die because she is 78 years old. One of the best-known facts of medical science—smoking kills—can't tell us whether a specific individual will die of smoking. About half of smokers die from smoking, but the other half do not.

Regression models also aren't very accurate at the extremes, precisely where we need them the most. Models can easily distinguish a 20 percent chance of death from a 30 percent chance of death, but they poorly distinguish 80 from 98 percent chances of death.[43] Many of us might well press on with painful medical treatments in the face of a 20 percent expected survival but focus on comfort rather than postponing death in the face of 2 percent expected survival. In other words, most of the results applicable to human decision making are clustered at the extremes, where regression models provide the least useful information.

These aren't just theoretical problems. Joanne Lynn and colleagues evaluated two large groups of patients in an elegant study in the 1990s: individuals who enrolled in the Study to Understand Prognoses and Preferences for Outcomes and Risks of Treatment (SUPPORT), and individuals in the APACHE III hospitals. Among SUPPORT patients, two weeks before death, most patients had a predicted 30 percent chance of living for at least six months. It wasn't until the day before death that people's chances of survival even fell below 10 percent. In the APACHE III database, those who died had a 14 percent chance of survival on the day before death and a 45 percent chance of survival one week before death.[44] It's almost impossible to know, even with the most sophisticated statistical techniques, that death is close enough for a living will to actually apply.

I've just described the cold machinations of statistical prediction scores. These are not the prognoses offered by physicians who actually know a patient. Surely we can do better by taking advantage of clinicians' medical expertise and intimate knowledge of their own patients.

The idea that people know better than computers has a visceral appeal: We humans have an instinctual suspicion of generality when it's applied to us. Regression models seem aloof and faceless, even hostile. We don't believe that a computer alone could know our future: A machine could never know how unique we are. Surely humans could do better than a machine.

Unfortunately, clinicians don't predict the future very well.[45] Even expert physicians commonly fall prey to typical cognitive biases. Researchers have found it distressingly easy to show that physician predictions can be manipulated by presenting strategic but irrelevant details.[46] While many clinicians think they know what to expect for a given patient, most of that optimism is driven by hindsight bias: After a particular outcome has occurred, we believe that we predicted what actually happened, even when we had predicted the opposite.[47]

In addition to being wrong, we human beings also tend to be over-confident. Physicians are highly skilled and perform certain tasks better than anyone else, but reality can get lost in the swell of self-assured expertise. Poor prognoses can serve as a defense mechanism. I've done it more times than I care to admit. If I say that survival is unlikely but we will press on, I look the hero when the patient pulls through. If I'm wrong in the opposite direction, all I can do is disappoint. It's not Machiavellian; it's a kind of unconscious reflex to avoid getting hurt. We clinicians don't just put on the show for patients, we do it for ourselves. It hollows you out as a healthcare worker to lose a patient that you expected to survive. So when in doubt, predict the worst. All of these factors contribute to the generally poor ability of clinicians to predict the future.

Researchers have put these questions to the test empirically. In general these studies follow a consistent methodology. Clinicians are asked whether they think a patient will survive her current illness. The more sophisticated studies ask for a specific estimate of how likely death is. A treating physician might say, "This patient will die" or "I predict a 70 percent chance of death for this patient." Estimates of this type from various doctors and nurses are then compiled over the course of the study period to see how accurate, on average, the predictions were. These studies have mostly demonstrated that healthcare workers—nurses usually more than physicians—tend on average to be more pessimistic than they should be when it comes to patients with life-threatening illness.

Sometimes this pessimism is strikingly out of proportion to reality. The elite Canadian Critical Care Trials Group studied a group of about a thousand patients, around a third of whom died. They discovered that ICU physicians were routinely too pessimistic. If physicians predicted less than 10 percent survival, 22 percent of patients survived, while if physicians predicted survival of 10 to 40 percent (less than even odds), fully four out of five (79 percent) survived. The only time the physicians gave accurate predictions was when patients were extremely likely to survive.

Nurses were even more pessimistic than physicians. When the nurses believed an individual had less than a 10 percent chance of surviving, nearly half actually survived.[48] According to this study, great news from your physician is great news, while bad news is uninterpretable.

In a study of experienced ICU clinicians in the United States, physicians almost always overestimated mortality. They performed best at predicting extremely low and extremely high probability of death, but failed more when the outcome was less certain.[49] A substudy of the SUPPORT trial suggested again that physicians were routinely more pessimistic than the statistical models and than reality.[50] Even where they do as well as the models, clinicians' accuracy is mediocre at best.[51]

Almost all of these studies have one important methodological problem. Unless physicians are extremely careful, their predictions can change the very future they are predicting. If physicians feel discouraged, they may communicate their hopelessness to patients and families. More than half of deaths—in some centers fully 90 percent—in the modern American ICU are preceded by a transition away from life-prolonging therapy.[52] Because the decision to allow a natural death by stopping life support is shaped by the expectations of physicians and families, doctors' predictions can become self-fulfilling prophecies.

Several years ago, I asked colleagues how severe shock had to be before treatment became pointless. Most said they knew they had reached a point of futility when they had to use a very high dose of adrenalin to boost a patient's blood pressure. Using this definition, I began to review the experience of all such patients at five hospitals over the course of five years. About one out of six of these patients survived. Among those who did not, we discovered that almost two-thirds died after a clinical decision—based on *futility*—was made to stop medical treatment. We have no idea what percent of these patients might have survived if the doctors hadn't decided to stop treatment.[53]

The inherent uncertainty of prediction means that in practice we have to impose some threshold for deciding when an advance directive applies. Does a 10 percent chance for recovery mean it's time to refuse further life support? A 1 percent chance? A one-in-a-million chance? Even the most sophisticated living wills use terms like "medical probability," "unlikely," or "very unlikely" without ever defining what those words mean.

When I describe the data about inaccurate survival predictions to colleagues, they often protest, "But what about the quality of life?" In other words, they believe that they are implicitly bundling death with survival with new disability. Even if some of the patients about whom they are pessimistic do survive, these patients must surely have a poor quality of life.

A group of researchers in Chicago who noted that physicians couldn't predict hospital survival well followed up their initial observation by examining longer-term outcomes among the hospital survivors. They found that of the 120 ICU patients for whom more than one clinician predicted death before hospital discharge, 112 died within six months. This group saw those later findings as the confirmation missing from their first study: To them, dead by six months was no different from dead in the hospital. The findings from Chicago haven't been confirmed yet; it's not clear whether this was another self-fulfilling prophecy (clinicians communicated their pessimism, so families and later clinicians made decisions to allow death to come sooner) or just physicians internalizing their long-term pessimism about outcome (they predicted death in the hospital because they expected death within a year). Crucially, this study and its interpretation do not acknowledge the fact that, to the patients, an additional six months of life may have been enormously meaningful to them and to their families.[54]

In general, predictions of disability are even less reliable than those for death. There is less experience with predicting the scope and nature of disability, and clinicians often struggle to distinguish their general pessimism from the specific questions about what life will look like after the ICU. In our research, among individuals with terrible shock who survived their stay in the ICU, no matter how sick they were in the hospital, disability was evenly distributed afterward.[55] So far, there isn't a reliable system for predicting the amount of disability a person will experience after surviving an ICU admission.

We've seen that physicians are often wrong when it comes to making predictions, including prognoses about the probability or timing of death. But living wills depend on the success of such flawed predictions; without accurate predictions by doctors, living wills won't work. Which means that they *don't* work. With so much uncertainty, a useful solution will have to be appropriately adaptable and sensitive to the uncertainty that will attend us as we struggle in the valley of shadows. It will need to honor us in our human specificity, both in the present and in the future.

BEING TRUE TO OURSELVES, NOW AND IN THE FUTURE

In Homer's *Odyssey*, the hero knows a thing or two about planning ahead. In the myth, Ulysses (*Odysseus* in the Greek) knows full well that he will not be strong enough to resist the sirens' wiles when his ship sails past them. But he can't bear the thought of not hearing their beautiful voices, so he has his sailors tie him to the mast and then stuff wax into their own ears.[56] By a conscious decision to bind himself in advance of events, Ulysses manages to navigate the temptation of the sirens safely.

Some people use this paradigm to aid decision making in modern life. A "Ulysses contract" is a form of precommitment they use to attain desired ends when they know they will be tempted to act against their better judgment in the future. You might agree to pay $100 if you smoke a cigarette or forget to go to the gym; or you might give your designated driver full authority to keep your keys no matter how hard you plead after you've had a couple extra drinks. Precommitment can be a powerful way to lose weight, exercise more, or avoid undesirable behaviors.

In medicine the best-known use of precommitment has been in mental illness, classically schizophrenia. Untreated, schizophrenia can be a horrifying condition in which sufferers live in crippling paranoia, unable to distinguish delusions from reality. Treated, schizophrenia can be compatible with a reasonably full life. But people with schizophrenia are notoriously prone to stop treatment, especially when they are feeling basically well. And when they are sick, they hate the treatments. Because society has a long history of violating the rights of the mentally ill, precommitment becomes a way to obtain consent during an episode of clear thinking for what doctors can do if the disease relapses or the patient loses insight into the need to continue medication.

But confronting death when it may be near isn't the same as worrying about eating too many cookies or forgetting to take your antipsychotic medications. While advocates think in terms of "precedent autonomy"—a way to provide informed consent well in advance of the time it is required—the law professor Rebecca Dresser places advance directives firmly in the category of precommitment strategies, not unlike

Ulysses contracts.[57] As precommitments, advance directives essentially stipulate, "If I or my family is tempted to keep me alive under difficult circumstances, don't. Even if it seems to them like the right thing to do at the time." Advance directives may become a promise that a person will not find a way through a new disability or challenge. (The special, rare case of permanent vegetative state shouldn't distract us from the much broader applications of living wills in practice.)

Crucially, people's preferences about how to confront life-threatening illness are quite fluid, making precommitment even riskier. By asking people the same questions at different points in time, researchers have found preferences for life-sustaining treatments unstable. Sometimes they would want life support, and sometimes they wouldn't.[58] The people who are most likely to be affected by advance directives are the ones most likely to change their minds about the instructions stipulated by those very directives.[59]

Precommitting to avoid wasting medical resources during serious illness is very different from being prepared to navigate a terminal illness or being supported during that final period of life. For terminal illness, what matters most is personalized guidance. The system is slowly improving its care of people who are wrapping up their lives, mostly through the fields of geriatrics and palliative care. These are the situations where palliative care really shines. Planning the shape of the final period of a progressive illness is much more about asking, "What phase of life am I in; what is coming up soon that I should prepare for?" than it is about asking, "Should I precommit to refuse a specific procedure in a hypothetical future state?"

Working through the problems of terminal illness with patients is demanding and important work. Guidance and support during serious illness is most useful and relevant when it is tied to actual circumstances and decisions to be made. Precommitting, through a living will, to resist the future temptation to waste medical resources draws attention away from where it matters: meaningful support during a health crisis. Living wills as such are generally so far separated from the actual course of events that they invite misleading speculation. When we are far separated from the actual decision to be made, we tend to rely on biases and misconceptions rather than intimate knowledge. The greater the separation between the decision and its application, the greater the likelihood that a kind of disability stigma may interfere with our thinking.[60]

"If I'm ever like that, let me die": Disability Stigma

Stacy, the rock climber described in the introduction, nearly died when her brother reported that she would never want to live as a paralyzed person. Commonly the question posed in precommitment strategies is whether to accept life with disability. But disability, as it turns out, isn't what most of us have thought it was.

It takes some time for a newly injured person to make peace with disability, but durable reconciliation generally occurs. Most disabled persons come to terms with despair and then find a meaningful life with the disability. People with disabilities know from personal experience how unbelievable it is at first that life can go on and how beautiful it is when life in fact does go on.

Disability makes sense only as part of a specific person's life. There's no real reason in general to favor the idea of paralysis or loss of limbs or mental impairment. Other things being equal, most people would rather be healthy than not. But as part of a particular person's life, those disabilities have a context in which they can be essential to the identity and beauty of an individual. In the context of a specific life, physical or mental disability can be powerful and worthy. Torn from that context, disabilities are only "disutilities" to be added to the debit column in a cost-benefit analysis.

The stigma of disability—the distaste most people have for limitations on health or abilities—is natural. But that stigmatization can cause us to make inaccurate decisions about our own possible future with disability. People who live with disability know only too well what it's like to have other people look at their lives with pity or revulsion. They recognize that if the onlookers could only inhabit their minds they would see the power and dignity that marks their life. These may be two cardinal rules about disability: Do not assume that a person can't adapt to new circumstances, and do not neglect the person within the disability.

The tension between the advance directives movement and disability rights has felt insoluble at times. Starting in the mid-1970s with

Section 504 of the Rehabilitation Act, American law began to recognize people with disability as a protected group with a shared identity, concerns, and rights. Disabled individuals came together and realized that the societal context of their physical struggles defined much of that disability.[61] They remembered that very recently many babies were allowed to die when they had congenital disabilities like Down syndrome. While others were precommitting themselves not to live with disability, the disabled had that life to live in a world of individuals who preferred death to life with disability. Antidisability messages were ubiquitous in society, but they were rapidly becoming impolite.

Emotions can run so high around this question that it's worth taking our time to think it through. Very few advocates of advance directives have ever been self-consciously opposed to disabled persons, and it's an uncomfortable thing to confess. I've had to acknowledge in myself in the last few years that I have at times been influenced by disability stigma in my treatment of disabled individuals in the ICU.

My intent is not to be inflammatory, but it's easy to miss a crucial point if we don't call a specific behavior by its name. The advance directive paradigm allows people to express disability stigma in a socially acceptable way because they channel it toward hypothetical future versions of themselves rather than any of their disabled acquaintances. But when people seek to understand what disability might be like for them in the future, they imagine what it would be like to be a disabled person, someone they know or have seen. There's no simple way around this fact.

As they are commonly applied, advance directives commonly ask people to break both of the basic rules of disability, with a subtle twist. The conceit behind living wills is that it's okay to embrace disability stigma as long as we're considering disability in our future selves. By asking us to see a future version of ourselves as disabled, we provide a space where we won't feel embarrassed or prejudiced if we stigmatize disability. But in general our only knowledge of disability comes from our distaste for frailty and dependence in the lives of others. While it is likely true that we know our future selves better than we know other people, many advance directives (those that apply to states other than permanent vegetative state) ask us to conceive of disability, abstractly, as separate from an actual personal identity and to also assume that we as individuals will not adapt to the new circumstance. And as we'll see in the next chapter, human beings are as remarkable in adapting to change—even negative changes like disability and loss—as we are limited in our ability to *imagine* that we will ever adapt well. Such failure of imagination is a major reason why advance directive are poor guides to life-and-death decisions; instead, timely guidance for choices made in real time, grounded in a person's actual health, is much more likely to lead to decisions that reflect our actual preferences rather than expressions of general disability stigma. Unfortunately, research demonstrates that this kind of timely guidance is thin on the ground when patients need it, and that living wills do not provide patients with choices that will be useful near the end of life.

WHEN THEY'VE BEEN STUDIED, LIVING WILLS DON'T WORK

Several important studies have addressed the empirical usefulness of advance directives and found them lacking. These studies date back to 1990, when the PSDA was passed and the Robert Wood Johnson Foundation funded a multimillion-dollar effort to demonstrate the utility of a kind of advance care planning.

A veritable Who's Who of medical, ethical, and legal experts assembled to design the SUPPORT study. Researchers enrolled seriously ill individuals who had been admitted to one of five hospitals. From its formal outcomes to its basic design, the SUPPORT paradigm assumed that people were undergoing expensive treatment near the end of life because either physicians and patients didn't understand how sick they actually were or there wasn't an extra nurse around to encourage communication if the physician or family were reluctant to talk. To test their hunch, researchers randomly assigned participants to receive or not receive access to the nurse-facilitator and for their physician to get a daily quantitative report of the chance of death during the hospitalization. Researchers decided that a DNR order early in the hospital stay was what should be measured to indicate effective change. Remember that at the time, physicians considered "full code" a moral failure and DNR the best marker of a good death.

The SUPPORT trial was entirely "negative," in the jargon of research studies: The study intervention was no better than doing nothing. The researchers and supporters of advance directives spent a decade trying to explain why the study failed to show an improvement. Their first interpretation was that more "proactive and forceful measures may be needed." In other words, just providing people support and information wasn't enough. They would need to be persuaded to behave differently. Remember the situation at the time: Doctors couldn't be trusted, bioethicists provided the outsiders' critical voice, and parents sometimes wanted to kill their own disabled babies. The adversarial, regulatory approach, with an eye toward wasted resources, clearly affected the conduct and interpretation of SUPPORT.

The failure of SUPPORT cast a pall over the field. Various other studies subsequently tested components of advance directives. A high-quality study led by the sociologist Peter Ditto specifically tested advance directives in a controlled experiment and found no benefit in 2001.[62] The accumulated evidence in favor of advance directives was poor enough that two ethicists called for the abandonment of living wills in 2004[63] and a 2008 report to Congress expressed profound skepticism about their usefulness.[64]

Then two studies appeared in 2010 that reportedly proved what other studies could not. One, conducted at a hospital in Melbourne, Australia, was an actual randomized study that included about 300 patients.[65] These Australian investigators were able to demonstrate that an intensive advance care planning intervention modeled on a US-based program led to less stress for families who had to decide on behalf of patients, although the effect on guiding treatment was less clear. The study was of higher quality than others, but included much more than living wills in the effort to improve care of individuals with serious illness. For unclear reasons, a review of data gathered for other purposes from the Health and Retirement Study made even bigger waves, despite being of lower quality.[66] An accompanying editorial even claimed that the study had somehow saved advance directives from oblivion.[67] Using a method that's susceptible to serious biases, the Health and Retirement Study results suggested that patients whose families remembered them as having completed some sort of advance directive were more likely to have died in a nursing home than in a hospital. This was only the best publicized of several similar studies.

With many studies showing no benefit and only one rigorous study, performed at a single hospital in Australia, showing benefit, there's just not enough empirical evidence to suggest that living wills work. If living wills were a medication, they would have been pulled from the market a long time ago.

The more powerful Physician Orders Regarding Life-Sustaining Treatment (POLST) documents are an even more complicated story. Several studies, especially of the Oregon experience, have suggested that patients with a POLST form tend to die in nursing homes rather than hospitals.[68] These results have been interpreted to mean that POLST forms work, but the studies require a look under the hood. They demonstrate that POLST forms tend to be enforced, not that they improve the expression of autonomy, align treatments with the individual's values and priorities, or improve the dying experience. Other studies suggest that POLST forms are often difficult for paramedics and emergency physicians to interpret, raising safety concerns about the central tenet of these forms—that they can be applied without the interpretation of an expert.[69] The much scarier question, whether patients actually agree with the preferences stated in their POLST forms, is just starting to be asked, and the experience with living wills suggests that the answer is unlikely to be reassuring. In my personal experience, I see them used as indiscriminately and hypothetically as living wills: commonly POLST forms require the opposite of what the patients say that they actually want.[70]

I'm aware that I have been harsh on advance directives here. I still agonize over how best to communicate my concerns about these documents. I admire the proponents of living wills; I am sympathetic to their ultimate desire to give an authentic voice to patients during health crisis. I think there are times when living wills can serve as conversation starters. The question is whether advance directives are tools in a toolbox that just needs a few more tools or whether advance directives are broken tools that can't yield their desired effect. Should we augment them or replace them entirely?

Everyone agrees that people want and need conversations and communication, respect and human flourishing, even in the face of impending death or other medical crisis. Advance directives, the disclosurist documents that support the appearance of autonomy, don't function well without substantial additional work. But here an important question arises. If advance directives do not function well on their own, what are they there for? It's reasonable to ask whether advance directives make the work that needs to be done easier in some way. If they did, that would justify augmentation rather than replacement.

So what is the work that needs to be done? Advance directives or something like them could be an important part of the natural process of dying. Phrased as they are—a vote in a referendum about national health policy expressed as precommitted responses to hypothetical future health states—I believe that they hurt rather than help. The problem is keeping people in the dark about what stands in their path of life, abandoning them when they are most vulnerable, failing to make the dying process as healthful and soulful as possible. Those problems are more important than squabbles about healthcare budgets. Fixing the human problems should be our highest priority.

Advance directives give people the hope that their voices will be heard. They make an implicit promise to speak for patients who cannot speak for themselves. Indeed, people have every right to demand that the medical system acknowledge them in their rich specificity. Yet by and large, living wills allow people to say YES! or NO! and little in between. Living wills, even the complicated ones, are rigid documents limited by their nature as precommitment contracts.

In the hospital, as elsewhere, people want to be known and honored in all of their distinctiveness and individuality. Our love of poetry or wild animals, the grueling battles we have fought with life, the crinkles in our foreheads or the tiny wetness of our kisses, distinguish us from others. So do our responses to the threats to health and the emotional turmoil that we confront during extreme illness. We want to preserve that personality in the face of life-threatening illness. Lasting solutions will need to replace one-size-fits-all advance directives with authentically personal alternatives. They will take careful research and understanding to avoid the errors of living wills. We don't yet have sufficient scientific knowledge to solve these problems meaningfully, but we could achieve it with careful, focused effort. Only then will the medical community have a hope of providing meaningful support for people as they make their way through life-threatening illness.

To be able to guide people through the valley of shadows, we need to better understand several elements of how human beings process information and make decisions. In chapter 4, we delve into the burgeoning knowledge about how the mind works and its implications for experience and decision making during life-threatening illness.

PRESENT

Chapter 4

Living Wills Don't Make Decisions;
Human Beings Do

Ken had emergency surgery for a tear in his colon caused by severe constipation. The bowel troubles came compliments of the oxycodone used to treat his chronic back pain, an increasingly common problem in American ICUs. Right after surgery, Ken had the moderate septic shock we typically see after a torn colon, but I was reasonably confident that he would recover well. Most patients do.

But a day later, Ken, still unconscious on the ventilator, developed a serious muscle injury out of the blue. It was detected in a routine blood test. We on the medical team struggled to understand what was going on; Ken's problem didn't fit into any of the standard categories for a muscle injury. We considered possible allergies to anesthetics or an autoimmune disease or even an adult-onset disorder of his mitochondria, the tiny cells-within-cells that provide the body its energy in usable form. I'd seen one or two of those rare mitochondrial disorders before, and it seemed possible that Ken fit the profile, albeit imperfectly. Ken's pattern of muscle damage didn't match anything any of us had seen before, though, and we were scratching our heads. Despite our uncertainty about the diagnosis and prognosis, we soldiered on, supporting Ken with our usual life support technologies.

Ken's wife Leslee was at the bedside in the ICU, on tenterhooks the entire time. The next step for diagnosis was a muscle biopsy in order to inspect the individual muscle fibers under a microscope. We consulted a surgeon so that we could get just the right muscle—the one that had looked most inflamed on a magnetic resonance imaging scan (MRI)—to give us our best shot at a diagnosis. The MRI also showed extensive swelling around the muscles and in the soft tissues. Just looking at the MRI pictures, without any other knowledge of Ken's situation, one could hypothetically propose that Ken was dying of massive infection of the thick white membranes, called "fascia," that cover human muscles.[1] And the radiologist dutifully raised the question in his report of the MRI.

Because those tissues wrap tightly around muscle but are not themselves supplied with much blood—they're sort of like plastic wrap made out of protein—they are occasionally susceptible to horrible infections. A few strains of *Staphylococcus* and *Streptococcus* bacteria have evolved a special cocktail of enzymes that chemically melt fascia. Once the microbes have liquefied the fascia, they spread throughout the body with stunning rapacity. The technical term for infection by one of these bacteria is "necrotizing fasciitis." Pronounced *fashy-itis*, the popular name for the condition is "flesh-eating bacteria." The popular name conjures in my mind a horde of microscopic wolves running amok, and the disease is, indeed, a horror to behold.

In the modern era of critical care, necrotizing fasciitis has become a treatable infection. Still, it remains a terrible diagnosis, generally requiring extensive surgery, possibly including amputation. When the infection is widespread, it can become absolutely untreatable. In those terrible cases, which are fortunately rare, we physicians risk disfiguring the bodies of our patients through multiple surgeries even as they die despite our best efforts.

The surgeon on call the day we needed Ken's biopsy was Dr. Jackson, a thorough and attentive physician. As he walked into our consultation, I didn't envy him. He was confronting an MRI that a hedging radiologist interpreted as consistent with necrotizing fasciitis, and a sick patient with a thick medical chart.

With a surgeon's focus, Dr. Jackson confirmed the radiologist's reading that the MRI probably showed necrotizing fasciitis throughout Ken's body. As an internal medicine doctor, stereotypically more prone to rumination than action, I tried to redirect Dr. Jackson to the reality of Ken's condition, which didn't remotely suggest necrotizing fasciitis. Ken's shock was getting better, not worse, his body showed no sign of new infection on bedside examination, and he had no risk factors for fasciitis. That the diagnosis was being discussed at all was based on the MRI report by the radiologist that included an exhaustive list of rare scenarios. Dr. Jackson resisted, though, and laid out a morbid sequence in which he would be required to remove all of Ken's limbs before Ken died regardless, his body disfigured beyond recognition. I told Dr. Jackson that such an outcome was extremely unlikely, but that if it were to be the case we could have a careful and honest conversation with Leslee at that point. But not before. We would only cause needless stress and pain by presenting this morbid fantasy as an actual possibility without any real evidence for it.

Surgeons have been taught over the last thirty years to emphasize every possible negative outcome of their surgeries when they speak with patients and families. It's part of the contemporary practice of informed consent that has resulted from disclosurism, probably combined with physicians' fear of lawsuits. These days, surgeons' notes include a talismanic recitation along the lines of: "Before proceeding to surgery, I warned the patient and his family of every possible complication, including infection, nerve injury, stroke, heart attack, bleeding, and death." True to the mandate of disclosure, Dr. Jackson recited the risks—both real and imaginary—of the muscle biopsy. Specifically, he told Leslee that he was worried about finding overwhelming infection at the time of surgery that would result in amputation of all limbs followed by inevitable death.

Knowing all too well the repercussions of a clinician's ill-placed words, I went to Ken's room right after Dr. Jackson left. I spent thirty minutes with Leslee and her son, reassuring them that the chances of a dire prognosis were remote. I explained that Ken's case could be disorienting or even frightening when doctors first reviewed his case. Slowly their agitation calmed.

In the event, a routine muscle biopsy that took a few minutes in the operating room showed no infection, just the swollen muscle we had expected. The relief was palpable, but Leslee struggled to rid herself of the aftershocks of the wild fear of Ken dying with all his limbs amputated.

Dr. Jackson had no idea of the psychological harm he had done to Leslee and her son. He seemed mostly glad he wouldn't have to mutilate

Ken as he died of necrotizing fasciitis. He went about his day, operating on other patients; he left a couple more notes in the chart and then disappeared from the case.

Dr. Jackson wasn't able to make the transition from an automatic response to the MRI report of the vivid possibility of fasciitis to thinking rationally about Ken's situation. The grotesque intensity of a rare diagnosis inflated its likelihood in his mind, a common mental error. He did his duty to disclose all possible dangers under the prevalent model of informed consent in medicine today. The conversation with Leslee thus represented a perfect storm of predictable cognitive errors and a poorly recognized moral hazard for physicians that's inherent in the contemporary medical system. Dr. Jackson did harm in the process, unaware of the meaning or implications of his actions. His irrational focus on flesh-eating bacteria created unnecessary misery for Leslee and her son.

Ken recovered, though he was discharged with substantial weakness and no certain diagnosis. He was glad to be alive and with Leslee, but we all ate the bitter fruits of Dr. Jackson's response to Ken's case.

This surgeon's response arose from the deep irrationalities that affect all human beings—expert and novice, physician and patient, specialist and generalist. I wish that the encounter with Dr. Jackson was an isolated case, but the reality is that similar irrationalities are ubiquitous in medicine, as in all of life. These irrationalities are critical to understand and address if we want to substantially improve the treatment of people with life-threatening illnesses. These irrationalities are a crucial reason why advance directives have failed to deliver on their promise.

THINKING LIKE A HUMAN BEING

We know a lot more about the specific limits of human rationality than we did four decades ago. In recent years, observations from marketing and cognitive psychology have coalesced into a formal scientific discipline founded by two psychologists studying economic behavior, Amos Tversky and Daniel Kahneman. In Nobel-prize-winning work, Tversky and Kahneman advanced conversations about human cognition and predictable irrationality to the point that some solutions are within reach; the findings are highly relevant to the path toward a humane ICU.[2]

These researchers pointed out the ways that researchers and policy makers have for many decades treated people as if they were superhuman, making perfectly rational decisions regardless of the circumstances. These researchers have led an assault on one of the linchpins of disclosurism. Their insights and criticisms are highly relevant to living wills and the problems of the modern ICU.

To solve the crisis that advance directives hoped to solve, we need to understand what it means to be *human*, not just in the sense of the aspirations and inherent dignity we possess, but the ways our brains mislead us. As people we are both magnificent and often irrational. The word "human" captures both of those meanings: We talk about human dignity to capture that magnificence, and we talk about being "only human" to acknowledge the limits to our ability to process information. By acknowledging the gaps in understanding we are all susceptible to, we can start to create strategies that will carry us through the valley of shadows with our human dignity intact.

The irrationalities that need to be navigated during life-threatening illness include the fact that we commonly employ automatic thinking that is efficient but inexact and that we fear both death and the chance that we might somehow be responsible for death. In each case, what matters is taking time to understand people in a way that is authentic to them as individuals. Neither perfect rationality nor unreflective irrationality represents the best solution to dealing with life-threatening illness.

WHAT YOUR BRAIN DOESN'T KNOW MIGHT KILL YOU

We are all human beings with human brains, and those brains operate imperfectly. Tversky and Kahneman proposed "heuristics" (simple rules of thumb) and "biases" (common errors in logic) to describe the systematic kinds of mental hiccups they and others observed in the psychology laboratory. Such errors ran the gamut from optical illusions to errors in estimating probabilities to holding frankly incoherent beliefs.

Cognitive psychologists and their kindred spirits in "behavioral economics" are trying to answer several questions: Why do humans not make the rational choices that economists and policy makers think they should? Why, in other words, do people buy things that aren't in their best interest? According to traditional economic theory, they should not, and yet they do, constantly.

They and others have suggested, metaphorically, that the mind can be divided into a fast, evolutionarily ancient but error-prone System 1, and a System 2 that provides the careful, logical reasoning that we associate with philosophers and mathematicians. In crude terms, System 1 is the impulsive jock (some people think of System 1 as the "monkey brain"), and System 2 is the scrawny nerd, both of them lurking inside all of us. In a manner of speaking, System 2 is the person the traditional economists wish we were, and System 1 is the person most of us are most of the time. Proponents call this the "dual process" theory of human cognition. The heuristics and biases are the currency on which System 1 operates.

The heuristics offer quick but often inaccurate solutions to complex problems. That they are fast is why we use them; that they sometimes give the wrong answer is a serious problem. The "availability heuristic" tells us that an event is more likely if we can easily remember an example of it.[3] If we've heard about a terrible accident with a toaster oven, we think of such ovens as more dangerous than they actually are. Terri Schiavo's excruciating plight on national television, like Nancy Cruzan's before her, sticks in people's minds. People may therefore refuse life support because they fear Schiavo's fate, even when such a fate is highly improbable. Alternatively, families may want to push hard if a friend survived some life-threatening illness in an ICU, even if the current patient has vanishingly poor prospects of recovery.

The availability heuristic affects physicians just as much as patients, and it may have caused Dr. Jackson to see flesh-eating bacteria when we asked him to perform Ken's muscle biopsy. It's possible that he lost a patient to the ravages of necrotizing fasciitis early in his career and thereafter tended to see it even when it was not there. I don't know about

Dr. Jackson's early career, but I do know that a painful experience with a patient's death may make a physician overestimate mortality among similar patients for years to come.

The brain saves time by applying heuristics like availability. Another time-saving device is to start from an initial estimate and then modify that estimate slightly, using the "anchoring and adjustment heuristic."[4] When the initial guess is close, we're in luck, but it's easy to start out with misleading anchors. Psychologists have repeatedly demonstrated how arbitrary the process is: Once we hear a specific estimate or number, we intuit that the truth must be somewhere near that number. How tall is the Empire State Building? If you just heard "2,000" you will guess close to 2,000 feet; if you just heard "500," you would guess more like 1000 feet. (Google says it's 1,454 feet, but that's beside the point.) If we have taken a stand in favor of a particular estimate, by saying it aloud or betting on it, our attachment to that anchor becomes much firmer. Anchoring can make people reluctant to stop life support once it has been started or to believe that survival is impossible after a rough night of setbacks.

These and other heuristics seem to me to be expressions of a broader phenomenon: Our minds seek and create coherence.[5] Even if we have to invent them, we look for or develop explanations that bring many pieces of information into agreement. As a result, we may identify patterns even when they aren't there. The simplest and best-known version of this false coherence is the "halo effect."[6] One impressive attribute leaves us thinking other attributes will be similar: Handsome people are more trustworthy, beautiful people are smarter. It's why pharmaceutical companies used to hire former cheerleaders as their salespeople: Doctors automatically trusted attractive, charismatic people. The human quest for coherence is much broader than the halo effect, though. "Confirmation bias"—accepting only information that fits with our preconceptions and discounting contrary evidence—is well known but still only one component of the tendency of human beings to create and maintain coherence.[7] We identify patterns, even nonexistent ones, and we use those patterns to understand complex phenomena. Characteristics can leak from one aspect to another as we build false coherence (a process some psychologists call "attribute substitution").

Availability and anchoring suggest the operation of false coherence, because we match our probability estimates to some external fact, even when that fact is entirely irrelevant.

This false coherence routinely muddles our thinking in the ICU. The ICU is so full of startling things that we often don't think clearly. We think with our reflexive System 1. For example, if an activity is painful, we think it's more likely to fail. If the activity is pleasurable, it is more likely to succeed. If a clinician likes or identifies with a patient, the clinician expects the patient to survive. And so on.

I failed through a kind of false coherence when I treated Jason, a schizophrenic man with a severe infection. When I first met him, Jason told me that he was unable to move his limbs and proved it to me by lifting his hands high over his head—"Doctor, I'm paralyzed." I suppressed a smirk and told him he was feeling weak because of the infection, a common symptom among people who have sepsis. I discounted Jason's report of weakness because of his schizophrenia and because he raised up his arms to prove to me that he couldn't move his arms. I filed him under "this is how a psychotic person experiences the weakness associated with sepsis."

It was a fair bet: The odds were definitely in my favor. That is, after all, the point of heuristics: They're usually good enough. Two days later, though, Jason was fully paralyzed from the effects of Guillain-Barré syndrome, a rare and devastating form of paralysis; he could no longer breathe on his own. Ashamed, I discussed Jason's recent history with his family in more detail after I connected him to the mechanical ventilator. They told me that he had been having about a week of progressing difficulty in walking and a sensation that his muscles weren't as responsive as they had been. The infection only came on the day he was hospitalized. The sepsis we were treating had nothing to do with his paralysis, which was in retrospect his main problem.

I should have noticed that I have a tendency to discount reports of symptoms from psychotic patients and should have recalled that most septic patients do not say that they are "paralyzed." I should have thought harder. But I didn't, and I failed Jason.

Heuristics and biases profoundly affect our ability to assess probabilities; this is where much of the most striking research has happened.

Even forgetting for a moment the fact that statistical models are bad at predicting the future for an individual patient, the basic reality is that most people, including doctors, are terrible at making judgments based on probabilities. Our human tendency to fall into cognitive traps and our rank inability to understand probability are especially threatening to one of the philosophical linchpins of the advance directive movement: our assessment, in the present, of our emotional response to a future state of affairs.

Affective Forecasting and Psychological Adaptation

Living wills ask us to consider future hypothetical health states and decide which of them are worse than death. Such judgments rely centrally on "affective forecasting," predicting how you will feel about a particular situation in the future. Unfortunately, people are terrible at affective forecasting—scores of psychology experiments have established that people have little idea how they will feel after an injury or new disability. Take one dramatic example, spinal cord injury. Many patients with acute paralysis from spinal cord injury want to die shortly afterward. Within a few months, most patients with spinal cord injury have adjusted to their new lives remarkably well, in spite of the challenges these injuries present.[8]

This is true in most of our lives. While we don't want to lose a job or a loved one, or develop a chronic illness, in general we make peace with changes that initially seem overwhelming. Daniel Gilbert, a psychologist at Harvard, has written eloquently about what he calls the "psychological immune system" to describe our remarkable resilience in the face of misfortune.[9]

I still remember putting my foot in my mouth when I met Rick and his wife. He had been paralyzed for twenty years when he came to my ICU with a bladder infection. Rick was delirious, so I asked his wife to supply the details of his medical history. I said, "So, other than the spinal cord injury, does Rick have any medical issues?" She stared back, uncomprehending. "Rick doesn't have any medical problems. What do you mean?" For Rick and his wife, his paralysis was just a part of life, like wavy blond hair, a square jaw line, or an endearing lisp. They no longer saw his paralysis as a health problem at all.[10]

The ability to adapt and incorporate disability into a meaningful, productive life is typical. The film *Million Dollar Baby*—in which the main character, a boxer named Maggie, becomes quadriplegic and has to decide whether to end her life—caused a stir among disabled viewers for just this reason. People living with paralysis knew all too well that Maggie's desire to commit suicide was almost certainly temporary. They knew that with time Maggie would very likely come to be glad she had survived. Such was the case with Stacy, the mountain climber who broke her neck in a climbing accident near Salt Lake City. But when decisions are made in the abstract, failures of affective forecasting distort judgments profoundly. We know that we would never want to live with paralysis because we have never been paralyzed and because we do not as a general rule know how we will feel in response to some future setback.

Amy Purdy, now a nationally prominent snowboarder, lost both legs to septic shock when she was 19. In her struggles to make sense of life without legs she moved through a state of despair, unable to get out of bed. Then she realized that the new situation, her life as "new Amy," allowed her to recreate herself. She could adjust her leg prostheses to be whatever height she wanted and could match the prosthetic feet to whatever shoes were most appealing in the department store.[11] While not every disabled person can aspire to Purdy's athletic accomplishments, her adaptability should be seen as a sign that we may be much more resilient after disability than we think.

Human adaptability in the face of disability matters because it's common to use the principles of health economics to motivate the use of advance directives. Health economists use surveys to arrive at quantitative measures of "quality of life," what they call "utilities." These measured utilities allow policy makers to compare, for instance, life with heart failure and diabetes to life with kidney failure. Where governments have to decide how to invest limited resources, they often do so in hopes of improving the quality of life. In simplest terms, a program that improves quality of life (increases utilities) will generally be higher priority than a program that does not. But the principles that govern decisions at the social level often don't make sense for the individual, precisely because the individual person will often adapt to the new disability. In this case, perspective is crucial to understanding how best to honor an individual patient. Unfortunately, the ominous shadow of death often makes it difficult to see matters clearly.

THINGS THAT GO BUMP IN THE NIGHT: THE SPECTER OF DEATH

Both death and our possible responsibility for death frighten us in ways that affect both decision making during life-threatening illness and the usefulness of living wills. This is a difficult topic, but it's crucial to confront it directly, because worry about death and our possible role in it may distract us so severely that we sink deep into our System 1 thinking.

Acknowledging our own mortality is generally frightening and painful. Some have argued that it is always utterly disorienting. While that is an extreme view, the intense distaste we generally feel at the prospect of conversations about death has to be admitted. Once we admit that we fear conversations about death, we can find ways through that discomfort. But the fear of death can hang about us like diffuse guilt, defying any attempts to think clearly.

Theories abound for why the topic of death disorients people. Freud is famous for his idiosyncratic theory about *Thanatos* (the Greek word for death), the death wish, which was a key to understanding our unconscious behavior.[12] Freud no longer commands much credibility as a scientific thinker about the mind, but his view of death as an unconscious fear that can drive us to distraction may still be useful.

Ernest Becker, a controversial mid-twentieth-century anthropologist, waged a battle against mainstream psychiatry as he moved from university to university, finally settling in British Columbia. Writing widely, if a bit erratically, he was particularly enamored of an on-again, off-again disciple of Freud named Otto Rank. Becker taught that the key to understanding evil and violence was that we are all unutterably scared of death. Both heroism and religion are manifestations of that unspeakable terror.

Becker was a talented writer, and he came at a historical moment that made his writing remarkably influential. He won a posthumous

Pulitzer for his 1973 *Denial of Death*, which summarized his basic theory that most of what is ugly in human behavior can be blamed on anxiety about death. With it, Becker spawned a school of psychology that experimented, inconclusively, with his ideas. Dressed up as "terror management theory," Becker's disciples report that in response to "mortality salience"—reminders that the person will one day die—subjects in psychology experiments tend to drive more recklessly, spend less carefully, and feel more heroic.[13]

In scientific terms, Becker's account is confused. He described universal human characteristics and blamed them only for evil, never for the good that humans do. Humans commit genocide, yes, but they also save others at considerable risk to themselves. Joseph Stalin was human, but so was Mother Teresa. Human beings were slavers, but they were also abolitionists. All of them were mortal, all susceptible to the disorienting influence of *Thanatos*.

Rather than provide elaborate accounts of "evil," others have seen mortality as a way of focusing our attention. The Stanford psychologist Laura Carstensen argues, with more nuance than Becker or Freud, that people become more "selective" when they believe their time is limited. When we feel that we have nothing but time, we have expansive thoughts and big aspirations. When we realize that our time is near its end, we tend to focus on relationships with our few close friends.[14] When my wife lost her eye to melanoma, I became a better husband and father. I started working more reasonable hours. I learned to cook and started doing dishes. I'm deeply embarrassed that it took the threat of my wife's early death to make me lead a mindful home life, but in my case it did. Many people find that the threat of death similarly focuses their minds on what matters. Still, even as the awareness of death can improve individual lives through greater regard for what matters most, it can also cause us to misperceive.

Becker was right about one thing, though: We don't like to confront death, and our discomfort in talking about death can create blind spots. Those blind spots affect both the individuals facing decisions and policy makers advocating change at the social level.

Take one straightforward example. Some researchers and policy makers concerned with medical treatment near the end of life cite large surveys that indicate that many people want to die at home.[15] Other things being equal, most people don't want to die in the hospital. I don't either. But those surveys do not capture what follows that thought in people's minds: "But if there's a chance I'll survive, please admit me to the hospital and give me that chance." To interpret the surveys in a way that is consistent with patients' actual wishes requires some nuance and attention to context.

Of course, other things being equal, most of us would like to die at home, at peace, surrounded by our loved ones in a comfortable bed. But most of us, unless we were already in the process of dying, would be willing to balance that desire against a meaningful hope of recovery from a specific illness. The balancing of those two wishes requires that we make compromises and acknowledge trade-offs; to do that requires attentive guidance over the course of serious illness.

There are always tragic trade-offs that must be confronted, but the general distaste for death can keep us from evaluating risks and benefits accurately. If, as a society, we push strenuously for everyone to die at home, at least some people will die much earlier than they would have otherwise, even when such an earlier death is not consistent with their honest, well-informed values and priorities.

The specific balance struck should appropriately vary from person to person. Some patients will feel that the risks of dying in the hospital outweigh the chance for longer life, while others will make the opposite assessment. If the goal is authentic personalization and self-determination, the relevant metric should be who would choose a given trade-off prospectively, not who died in a hospital. Even the prior sharp boundary between death in the hospital and death at home is blurring recently, as more and more ICU and hospice clinicians help dying patients who desire it to get home for their last hours, days, or weeks.

Fear of death isn't the only burden that short-circuits our thinking. Human agency plays an important role here too. Agency is the idea that a person is the cause of something. We exercise agency when we choose, when we act in the world. As self-determination, human agency is the foundation of much of modern political and moral philosophy. Self-determination is appropriately cherished.

But agency is often deeply painful when it comes to deciding about death. Before the advent of modern medicine, while most people resisted the prospect of death, it wasn't really up to anyone to decide when a specific individual would die of natural causes. That changed dramatically with the advent of modern ICUs. Their life support technologies weren't just a medical marvel, they introduced human agency into a situation where that agency can be crippling. There wasn't any real choosing to die before, just electing to make peace with the fact of death. What had been a question of Nature or the will of God—whether or when a particular person was in fact dying—came instead to be a matter of human judgment. With the move away from medical paternalism, that choosing fell increasingly on people with no training or experience.

In the past, people thought of God as the agent responsible for important events. "Providence" was the term to describe God's agency in human history. In contemporary society we still occasionally hear an echo of that old providentialism in phrases like "Everything happens for a reason." The time in any individual life when Providence mattered most was the timing of death. For most of human history the deathbed was fundamentally about aligning one's life and will with the dictates of Providence.[16]

A paradox lurks within advance directives. On the one hand, human agency matters a great deal. On the other hand, people want to be able to make peace with inevitable death when the time comes. As a result, agency and Providence often work at cross-purposes. Agency places responsibility squarely in the hands of the individual, while Providence places responsibility outside the individual.

Agency has been welcomed by ethicists and most people in most of their lives, but it has remained unwelcome at most actual deathbeds. The advantage to Providence is that people don't need to see themselves as causing death, whereas with agency people often see themselves as responsible for death. Many researchers have demonstrated this fact, both in lab experiments and in the real world. Most people do not want to feel responsible for a death. The prospect of feeling responsible may seriously complicate medical decisions. Qualitative research has shown that people prefer not to experience potentially tragic medical decisions as decisions but rather as making peace with the inevitable.[17] Elegant work in neonatal ICUs has demonstrated that feeling responsible for a decision to stop treatment induces substantial distress.[18] Advance directives force people to treat those experiences as decisions, even when seeing them that way is foreign to their actual sensibilities.

Life support technologies introduce agency into many deaths, whether we like it or not. That agency is here to stay. The question is how best to deal with agency and death. Under paternalism, the physician absorbed the agency surrounding death without comment. That process stole from patients and families not just the burden of tragic decisions but also the chance to be heard and respected in their individuality and opportunities to make peace with death while wrapping up their lives. A rigid interpretation of advance directives, with their focus on procedures and anticipated hypothetical decision points has mostly placed a bewildering burden on people without providing tools to make sense of that burden or any guidance in wrapping up their lives.[19] Even something as simple as a frame shift could help—rather than asking for opinions about hypothetical procedures, clinicians could clarify with people what phase of life they are living and what might be the clues by which they will know that their time has come. A focus on procedures reflects the bias of clinicians, the "medical industrial complex," and culture warriors; an emphasis on phase of life and understanding the signs that a life is wrapping up would be more relevant to how people actually experience their lives and the course of illness.[20]

Crucial to guiding patients and families through the valley of shadows is learning how, in a way that is true to patients as individuals, to reconcile with death when that time comes. That capacity is something our culture has largely lost, and that loss has made it difficult to see clearly. As we work to improve the experience of life-threatening illness, we have to grapple with how best to approach these transitions. It's not an insoluble problem, but it requires that we confront our irrationalities as individuals and as a society. Careful attention to clinicians' biases is critical to navigating the spaces between fighting for life and reconciling with death.

MORAL DISTRESS CAN BLIND CLINICIANS

Discomfort with death and anxiety about agency mold clinicians' responses to their patients. Health professionals in the ICU are just as human as the patients and families they treat. Clinicians bear a variety of cognitive biases and blind spots that shape their interactions with patients and families. Advance directives may worsen those blind spots by creating a serious moral hazard for clinicians. The hazard is made possible by a combination of moral distress and failures of situational awareness—the ability to step outside a situation to see beyond blind spots—that afflict health professionals across the spectrum from hospital executives and ultraspecialist physicians to orderlies and everyone in between. That unfortunate circumstance has caused many of us healthcare workers to betray our higher natures.

When I talk with medical students and especially physicians-in-training about code status, they tend to grimace, frown, and squirm in their seats if I ask them to think about the last time they performed CPR. They often find it difficult to articulate precisely what bothers them. They feel that it's "wrong" or "cruel" or "terrible," but it's hard for them to say why exactly. When we talk the problem through, they tend to realize that they are framing CPR as an assault on a dying person. If they are feeling pessimistic, they see the person as dead at the time they begin CPR. I understand their distress; every time CPR fails to resuscitate the individual (and it fails more often than not), they feel more certain that CPR is something cruel you do to a dead person. And decent people do not assault the dead. Once you frame CPR that way, you're going to hate it.[21]

But the clinicians' view may be light years away from how a patient and family might perceive CPR. In fact, it's pretty clear that patients and families in general do not think CPR is either wrong or cruel. When the patient survives well, everyone is delighted. When the patient doesn't survive, and sometimes that death comes after a brief period of unconsciousness, families are often grateful that the physicians tried to prevent death. The main exception is when the individual was already dying from a terminal illness at the time of cardiac arrest.

The actual data on CPR are reasonably clear: In general one in seven patients survives in-hospital CPR with satisfactory neurological outcomes.[22] Physicians commonly understand this to mean that most CPR is futile. But many patients would be willing to undergo CPR for a one in seven chance of survival when the alternative is immediate death, *as long as* they are not forced to stay alive in a vegetative state or feel that life is already near its end. You don't need to be pathologically afraid of dying to say that you would be willing to try a rescue option that could save you from certain death one time out of seven.

Epidemiologists and clinical researchers use a single statistic, the number-needed-to-treat (known as the "NNT" in the jargon), to define the success of a medication or a procedure. The number-needed-to-treat is the answer to the question "How many patients need to be treated with a medication before one of them who would otherwise have died will live instead?" A drug that worked as well as CPR (treat seven patients and one will survive who would not have otherwise) would be a blockbuster beyond anyone's wildest imaginings. Nobel prize medals and Wall Street fortunes would follow such results. Most drugs that the Food and Drug Administration (FDA) approves are an order of magnitude less effective than CPR: Many have a number-needed-to-treat in the 500–1000 range. Few treatments we commonly employ in medicine are as effective as CPR.[23]

So why would physicians and social commentators strenuously reject a treatment that is so successful? This odd situation comes from confusion about context. In some patients, especially those with advanced terminal illness before the cardiac arrest, CPR is much more likely to deform a death than to save a life. But that is not an attribute of CPR, it's a feature of a given person's phase of life. Once again, the procedural focus of advance directives drives attention away from where it belongs. Any discussions about CPR should primarily concern an individual's present level of health, phase of life, and general life philosophy, not the attributes of CPR per se. And, critically, people should not be forced to remain in a vegetative state merely because they once consented to CPR. To frame the question as if what matters is whether CPR is undertaken, rather than what should happen if CPR fails, is to create a false dichotomy that interferes with self-determination.

The distaste that students, trainees, and, frankly, most healthcare professionals feel toward CPR can be thought of as moral distress, the emotional discomfort associated with feeling forced to violate one's convictions. While no one experiences that moral distress quite as vividly as young doctors starting their careers, all of us are susceptible to it.

Clinicians' antipathy for CPR routinely spills over into how they communicate with families. I still occasionally hear physicians ask patients "When you die, should we break your ribs and shove a tube down your throat?" in order to determine code status. I asked that question myself many times earlier in my career. Well-meaning physicians, squeamish about CPR, thereby pressure patients to approve a Do Not Resuscitate/Do Not Intubate (DNR/DNI) order. Alternatively, they may force a false dichotomy: be DNR or have everything done, no matter how painful. In the right situation, it's not wrong to invoke respect for the dead or distaste for uncomfortable procedures in explaining why CPR doesn't make sense for a specific individual, but the attributes of the patient are what matters, not the attributes of CPR. Specifically, there are certain phases of life when CPR may interrupt a natural dying process that would otherwise be welcomed. Most patients dying of advanced cancer would not want CPR if they were fully informed. In such a case, despite its vividness in the minds of clinicians, the question of CPR or other specific life support procedures is only one small part of the important conversations about how to live life's final chapter.

Moral distress isn't a small problem. For physicians and nurses, such distress is strongly associated with burnout, depression, substance abuse, and professional disengagement. Moral distress is a problem that needs to be confronted and resolved, both to help clinicians and, most importantly, to align treatments with the needs of patients.

The death of patients we had hoped would live is a painful burden. I am sad when any of my patients departs life. I'm not sad because death represents a medical failure, and I don't let the sadness force me to apply high technology indiscriminately. But, turning to the words of the poet John Donne, I feel hollowed out when another human being dies. The figurative tolling of the bell to mark a patient's death is a sound that pierces me with loss. We humans are beautiful things, and our departures deserve to be mourned. But the sadness that we clinicians feel must not drive us to make irrational decisions that harm our patients.

Discomfort with death also keeps many clinicians from realizing that—because they must treat patients before they know whether the given patient will live or die—their care for those who die is *part of* their care of those who survive.

Sometimes ICU clinicians have to provide treatments that, in retrospect, may seem useless. It's a simple matter of numbers. Realistically our sickest patients probably have about an 80 percent predicted mortality with treatment and a 100 percent predicted mortality without treatment. In our study of very severe shock, a condition some physicians viewed as futile, we saw about a 20 percent survival. With this spread—80 percent treated and 100 percent untreated mortality—the difference between untreated and treated cases means that four out of five catastrophically sick patients will not survive no matter what we do. But one of the five, a person who would otherwise have died, will survive. At the time we provide treatment in the ICU we rarely know which outcome awaits the specific patient. We have to make peace with that uncertainty, but it's emotionally wrenching to treat a patient who ultimately dies. The pain of losing four people can be so intense that clinicians are inclined to stop treatment. When that happens something—someone—will be needlessly lost. Strenuous and diligent work for the other four is part of the offering we bring to the one.

We must never inflict treatments on people who would not want them, and we must not use the four patients who do not survive as "experiments" for the one person who does. But we can't know beforehand what will happen to an individual patient, so we press on, with permission, with what seems fair to all five and consistent with their values. We can dedicate our work and anxiety on behalf of the four who die—as long as we responsibly support them and their families in honesty and compassion—to the ultimate recovery of the one.[24]

As long as ICU treatments are respectful, desired, and personalized, clinicians can understand the distress they feel at death and the miseries of the ICU in a new light. With current understandings, when a patient dies clinicians may be left only to regret that they attempted life-saving treatments; by understanding the interconnections among patients, the emotional pain of treating those who ultimately die can be consecrated on behalf of those who live. This awareness must not decrease the quality of end-of-life care for anyone, but should help clinicians see their labors in the valley of shadows as a source of hope rather than distress.

Cardiopulmonary resuscitation is only the most dramatic of the procedures that give clinicians pause. They can just as easily feel distress about other life support therapies when they feel that the chances of recovery are low. Given that doctors and nurses routinely overestimate mortality, a cognitive error made worse when they are distressed, this moral distress can lead us away from authentic autonomy.

Research confirms that the moral distress of the physician—far more than the specific values of the patient or family—drives the application of advance directives in real life.[25] Advance directives thereby become a method by which treatments that physicians find distressing will not be provided to patients, even if the patients would benefit from them and want to receive them when fully informed. As advance directives evolve into increasingly detailed lists of life-sustaining therapies, physicians' moral distress may become even more influential.

LIVING WILLS CREATE A SUBSTANTIAL MORAL HAZARD

The term "moral hazard" refers to aspects of a system of incentives that may encourage people to act inappropriately. Classic examples of moral hazard are well-intentioned regulatory schemes that accidentally encourage pollution, insider trading, or faulty mortgages. In healthcare, the traditional method of compensating physicians and hospitals is a typical moral hazard: Doctors are paid to do anything; they aren't paid to do the *right* thing.

In the case of advance directives the moral hazard has three main components.

First, advance directives encourage clinicians to think solely in terms of procedures to refuse. The procedural focus distracts from what matters, life's meanings when death may be near. Life is about more than just deciding at what moment we breathe our last. It's about making the best of life as we live it, including its final phases. Clinicians tend to forget about the burdens borne by survivors and the deformation of dying that can occur regardless of which medical procedures are selected or declined. Instead of instructions along the lines of "Don't keep me alive if you're feeling pessimistic," people need a way to communicate "Walk with me, honestly and attentively, when death may be near" and expect that clinicians will honor that wish.

Second, by pretending to provide meaningful instructions to physicians while doing nothing of the sort, living wills encourage overinterpretation and overapplication. Multiple studies have shown that, contrary to the actual desires of patients and families, physicians and nurses often take orders of DNR/DNI to mean that they should limit many other life-prolonging treatments. Some people call this "indication creep," and it's very common.[26] I've lost count of the times that trainees have decided that a patient who only wanted to reject permanent vegetative state has in fact refused all life-sustaining measures under any circumstances.

The advance directives system, as with so much of disclosurism, does not and likely cannot provide the information and expertise people need to direct their medical treatment. Most individuals have a reasonable sense of their values, goals, and priorities, but they don't know how to map those specifics onto technical medical decisions. What people need and want are guides who know them well and help them walk their own path through life-threatening illness.

Third, by placing the burden of navigating life-threatening illness squarely on patients and families, living wills encourage physicians to abdicate their responsibility in this emotionally and morally fraught area. In Jodi Halpern's insightful terms, physicians' "own unacknowledged fears of loss and death serve as a barrier to emotional engagement with patients facing death and dying."[27] The strong focus on a specific, narrow view of autonomy and its advance directives has left many physicians reluctant to contribute to conversations about aggressive therapy near the end of life, either deferring or squabbling with families rather than seeking out ways to accompany people through their experience of life-threatening illness. These physicians are not lazy or callous; as human beings they find conversations about life's end difficult, even painful. The advance directive fosters the illusion that a few checkboxes on a legal form constitute sufficient response to patients' needs during life-threatening illness. However unconsciously, many of us clinicians seem to hope that we will be liberated from a painful duty if we can just hand a disclosure document or "code status" form to patients, thereby avoiding the more complicated and stretching work of walking attentively with people through life-threatening illness.

By pretending to be a solution to an important problem, advance directives distract us from actual solutions. People need guides through the valley of shadows, not a form listing medical treatments they would reject under hypothetical conditions. The old parentalism was a broken system, but so is the style of autonomy that replaced it. Patients and families need more from clinicians than a clipboard with an advance directive on it. People need health professionals to know their values and priorities, to speak openly and honestly with them, and to help them understand how to translate their priorities onto the array of possible medical decisions that exist. That process is much harder on physicians than advance directives. Physicians need to take the risk and bear some burden, not to overshadow the patient's autonomy but to enhance it.

I was a physician-in-training when I met Judy and her son Tim, a thirty-eight-year-old trying to reboot his life. Tim had achieved a year of sobriety after two decades of severe alcohol addiction. But as his terrible luck would have it, he developed a bleeding ulcer that led to cardiac arrest when the blood pouring from his stomach closed off his windpipe. Judy, who had stood by Tim his entire life, shook visibly as she told me how the emergency room doctors just barely got his heart beating again. Within about twelve hours of his arrival in our ICU, Tim was almost brain dead.

He had always made it clear to his mother that he would never want to live as a "vegetable." Judy wanted to be true to her son's life philosophy, but she couldn't bear the thought of stopping life support therapies. After we had made the difficult decision to allow a natural death, Judy found me at the nurse's station and said, "I can't do this without you, Dr. Brown. I have to rely on you. I need you here for the whole process."

It was one of the first times someone had put such explicit trust in my predictions. I had done my duty to her by reporting the prognosis and the medical options. I didn't want to also bear the burden of the decision. It frightened me to realize that Judy's decision ultimately depended on my input. I went back to the senior neurologist and my ICU supervisor and made absolutely sure that we were unanimous in our predictions about Tim's prospects. When the sad answer didn't change, we proceeded to honor Tim's life philosophy and stopped life support therapies. I held my arm around Judy's shoulder and felt her convulse with tears as Tim slipped from life.

The experience stretched me; I was exhausted for days. I realized on a personal level just how much I had allowed the focus on autonomy to place the emotional burden of critical illness entirely on patients and families. Even though everyone agreed that the right decision had been made, I had been more than happy to impose the full force of agency on Judy. That general approach had made my life a lot easier: I pretended that my prognostications weren't having a major influence on decisions. I just turned the stress over to the patients and families and went about my workday.

This behavior is supported by the pretense that advance directives are driven by patients rather than physicians. They encourage clinicians to work from a menu of morbid-sounding medical treatments from which they ask patients to choose. "Would you like your ribs crushed," the waiter asks, "or perhaps a tube shoved down your throat like a blunt fish hook?" Instead of a menu, though, patients need an experienced guide to help them make their way along a technically complex and morally exhausting path. The guide does not require perfect foresight but must be ready to meet patients and families on their terms, to know what tends to happen in similar medical circumstances, to be able to help patients and families map their convictions and personalities onto the difficult choices that confront them.

WE MUST CHOOSE TO SEE

Working to avoid the moral hazards rampant in current decision making in the ICU is part of a much larger quest for situational awareness.[28] Clinicians, like everyone else, make cognitive errors. In fact, as professionals we are prone to an extra set of errors related to our special expertise.[29]

Some errors are mistakes in diagnosis. Recall that heuristics are efficient rules to get close to the truth in common circumstances. Recognize a familiar pattern and give it a familiar name. This woman with anxiety disorder says she can't breathe? She's having a panic attack, not a pulmonary embolism. While a panic attack may be more common, occasionally people with anxiety have a blood clot in their lungs.[30]

The development of expertise, such as is possessed by clinicians, creates a special kind of blind spot. As we become expert at something, it becomes automatic. We perform without specific attention to the task at hand. It's the basis for the phrase "practice makes perfect" and the concept behind the "10,000 hours" notion popularized by Malcolm Gladwell.[31] This training into automaticity is how concert pianists can move their hands across a piano too fast for anyone to really know where the fingers are at any given moment, including the pianist herself.

But this strength of expertise can easily become a weakness. We lose track of changing conditions that can make our automatic, expert response precisely the wrong answer. We as human beings can get so locked into automatic thinking that we miss the big picture or new, critical information.

Physicians develop expertise in making diagnoses and in performing procedures. I have seen tragic deaths result when physicians are unable to move from their automatic routines to better-informed observations. A middle-aged woman has pain at the bottom of her rib cage on the left. A cardiologist performs a catheterization to be sure it is not a heart attack, which it isn't, so he sends her home. She bleeds to death the next day when the aneurysm in her spleen ruptures. The cardiologist had put the patient in the "make sure it's not a heart attack" basket and hadn't asked why the pain was closer to her spleen than her heart.

As Albert Mulley and Glyn Elwyn, two physician pioneers of shared decision-making, have argued persuasively, similar diagnostic errors can prevent clinicians from understanding who patients are and what they actually want. Failures to diagnose a patient's values and priorities are susceptible to the same cognitive errors as medical diagnoses and are just as important.[32]

Beyond diagnosis, the two main problems that physicians fall into are errors of prognosis and pseudo empathy. These problems are often intertwined.

From studies we know that errors of prediction are common; prediction is almost certainly even less accurate in the real world where researchers aren't watching.[33] Clinicians tend to misunderstand their patients' priorities and, when they discuss prognosis, to overestimate adverse outcomes if they believe that an individual's quality of life is poor. In the cancer world, it's the opposite problem. There, physicians are predictably too optimistic.[34] I suspect that the reason for this opposite effect is that cancer patients are awake and talking, while patients in the ICU are often unconscious. It is too painful to picture someone you can speak with as dying; it's much easier to conceive of a person on life support systems as dying. Here false coherence makes yet another appearance: Irrelevant but evocative information shapes our understanding of other facts, profoundly.

Crucially, clinicians don't realize that they are making errors of prognosis. Nor do they realize that their thresholds for assessing likelihood (what is reasonable, 1 percent, 5 percent, or 10 percent chance of survival?) may differ substantially from their patients'. Basic errors of prognosis get worse in the presence of moral distress. A positive feedback loop develops, driven by what psychologists call pseudo empathy. Pseudo empathy is another example of false coherence, in which the clinician imagines that she understands how the patient feels because the patient's feelings must be the same as her own.

Studies suggest that physicians and especially nurses actively dislike providing advanced medical care to people with severe disability or those that seem hopeless. Burnout makes it worse, especially for nurses.[35] I have experienced those feelings, too, sometimes acutely. I'm not proud of that fact, but it's true. My gut tells me that it is true of every single clinician at some point. The pain we healthcare workers feel at running life support for people who may not benefit colors our thinking about the chance that the treatment will be successful. It also keeps us from seeing what is most consistent with the actual patient's goals and aspirations.

My practice now when I'm working through questions about life support with families and patients is to ask myself whether I am feeling moral distress. Is the patient different from me? Does she remind me of a negative experience I've had? Is he disfigured in some way? Am I in a bad mood? Is a conflict at home leaving me feeling unsettled? If I detect any moral distress, I pause and reassess before providing input about prognosis. When I have significant doubt, I reach out to a colleague who can act as "designated driver," a method I've employed in high-risk medical procedures for years. That designated driver isn't performing the procedure, she is watching it from a distance to notice what those engrossed in performing the procedure cannot. This same technique is useful for morally charged discussions about when or whether to allow a patient to die.

A colleague recently approached me about what to do with Brad, who was suffering with uncontrolled high blood pressure and a blood-clotting disorder. He had suffered multiple strokes and was now facing the loss of an arm because a new blood clot shut off all blood flow near the armpit. Before all the problems with blood clotting, Brad had an embarrassing prescription drug habit. The reality, as sad as it is to admit it, is that many people saw Brad as a deadbeat, unlikely to contribute meaningfully to society even before the crisis that brought him to our ICU. As is common after a stroke, Brad couldn't participate in conversations because he was delirious. He seemed to change his mind twice an hour about what he wanted done—to die or undergo amputation—but could barely keep his attention on anyone for more than twenty seconds.

My colleague consulted me to talk the case through, and it became apparent that his visceral response to Brad was limiting his situational awareness. My partner inferred from Brad's troubled social status that he would not want to live with the stroke and amputation. I became my colleague's designated driver, as he had been for me in other cases. We saw that an irrelevant detail—the stigma of drug addiction—was clouding the decision-making process. Brad had his surgery, and he ultimately recovered well. If anything, the brush with death brought him clarity. He got a job, became independent, and is flourishing despite the amputation and the stroke.

Failures of situational awareness are often quite predictable. The people with the least reliable information may on average be the most certain of their views. Physicians almost always speak from remembered experience. Smaller hospitals don't have much experience with really sick patients. This means that in the smaller hospitals physicians and nurses will have limited exposure to extremely sick patients who go on to survive. The patients they treat are the ones they don't transfer to larger hospitals, for whatever reason. But the usual reason not to transfer a sick patient is because the patient was ready to die. Thus, when these clinicians try to process the likelihood that a given patient will survive a terrible illness, they tend to be very pessimistic. Those of us who practice in larger, referral center hospitals are accustomed to caring for the sickest of the sick. We know from studies that only about one in three or one in four of those really sick patients referred to us will die, on average. And there's the disturbing word from psychology that our confidence may be inversely proportional to our actual knowledge.[36]

I still remember Evan, a middle-aged man transferred from a small hospital to our referral center "to die." He came to the original hospital with septic shock, infection so severe his body couldn't maintain its blood pressure in a healthy range. A couple of tests suggested that he had infection in the blood, even though his main problem was a severe pneumonia. An ultrasound of the heart showed some ominous-looking shadows near one of the heart valves. At that point the referring physicians told Evan's family that he was as good as dead. No one, they said, could survive an infected heart valve that resulted in shock.

Evan's family demanded that he be transferred to a larger hospital. Our team would either offer Evan another chance or confirm the death sentence. His family looked like cornered mountain lions when I first met them, full of fear and rage, as they waited for me to say that Evan would soon die. I told them I couldn't give an answer right away. We repeated the heart ultrasound, sent new blood tests, watched him for a day, and requested all of the records from the referring hospital. The more I looked, the happier I felt for Evan and the sorrier for the anxiety his family had needlessly suffered. The results suggesting blood infection were false positive—bacteria from skin that hadn't been sufficiently cleansed before the blood sample was drawn. And the infection on the heart valve that the ultrasound had suggested was just a bunch of static on the image. I returned to his family with the results of my review: About 85 percent of patients like Evan survive. Evan's family was intensely relieved, and he recovered well after another three days in our ICU.

Evan would have met a living will's usual criteria for letting him die at the smaller hospital. He was unconscious and his treating physicians believed that they were only prolonging the process of dying. Evan did not himself have a living will; if he had had one and his family hadn't protested, he might have died.

I've had patients transferred over the vociferous objections of the referring physician because they are doomed to die, when the patient only ever had about a 25 percent chance of death by objective criteria. Of course, a one in four chance of death is not to be trifled with; the needs of the one who goes on to die must be met, compassionately and authentically. But making people believe that they will certainly die when they will likely survive is wrong, however sincere the conviction.

The threats to clear thinking are important for everyone involved in an ICU encounter. Unchecked, these problems can lead to decisions that do not represent the autonomous desires of patients. A key question is whether advance directives do anything to limit these risks. The stark reality from my observations and the scientific literature is that in fact they may make these problems worse.

The disclosurist framework leads physicians to feel that their responsibilities only stretch as far as the question of whether to use life-prolonging treatments. The system may thereby worsen clinicians' blind spots regarding human priorities near the end of life, the final tasks that can be so deeply healthful when it is our time to go. I witnessed this failure firsthand in the case of my grandfather, Howard Morris, whose opportunity to say goodbye was stolen from him as surely as anything can be stolen.[37]

Howard was a retired food biochemist at the University of Minnesota, the "father of the American *bleu* cheese" according to people in the know. He was physically vigorous—a semiprofessional golfer and avid rock collector—until the onset of Parkinson's disease at age 81. He moved into an assisted living facility after the Parkinson's made it difficult for him to walk independently. He was stoic but visibly frus-trated with his physical disability. A slip and fall in the bathroom at his facility landed him in the hospital. The fall caused a large bruise deep in his brain.

When he entered the hospital, Howard was wide awake with no real symptoms except for a minor headache. The pain improved after a dose of extra-strength Tylenol. A practical, detail-oriented scientist, Howard had always known what he wanted from the medical system, which was not to prolong artificially the process of dying. He was adamant to the physician who admitted him to the hospital that he would never want life support or even brain surgery. The consulting neurosurgeon heard that statement as permission not to operate because the "patient declines aggressive care." My grandmother and uncle understood the doctors to be telling them that Howard had suffered a "small stroke," which is what they told the rest of the family. The report of a small stroke, what I assumed was just a "transient ischemic attack," didn't indicate alarm to any of us, though I had been wanting to fly to Minnesota to see him for several months. I decided, almost on a whim, that a minor hospitaliza-tion should be cause enough to see my favorite grandparent. I booked a flight for the weekend, just a few days away.

I left the hospital after an overnight shift and went straight to the airport. By the time I arrived in Minnesota, I was tempted to take a nap in the rental car before seeing Granddad. But a nagging feeling drew me to the hospital without delay. I expected to catch up on life with my grandfather: He loved to talk about experiments, the scientific method, and his distrust of weepy people. He liked that I also loved science. Instead of our usual conversation, though, I found Granddad deeply unconscious, breathing in a pattern of accelerating panting followed by stretches of no breathing at all.[38]

I called for the resident, who was visibly panicked. Although he wasn't at the bedside when I arrived, he had been nervously calling for the cavalry after the nurse told him about Howard's irregular breathing and coma. He wanted me to locate and review my grandfather's living will. "Are you sure he's DNR/DNI?" he asked. I hadn't actually seen the living will, although I knew my grandfather well enough to know that he wouldn't want life support at this stage of his life.

The resident's nervous tension was contagious, and I found myself troubleshooting medical details with him. It took long minutes to discover that instead of a small stroke, he had a bloody bruise located in a part of the brain that often causes swelling. I started to wonder whether it would be okay to put a small drain through Granddad's skull to allow him to awaken long enough to be able to talk to me again. I ached at seeing him in that hospital bed, so much like a corpse and so little like the man who had mentored me from boyhood on. I wanted to yell and cry at the same time.

After some hectic minutes rushing about, we all agreed that Howard was actively dying, would not have wanted aggressive medical treatments, and that we should call my grandmother and uncle to bid him farewell. Granddad died about twenty minutes later, as the pauses between the cycles of panting lengthened into a final agonal shudder. His chest stilled, and the color of life drained from his face.

I couldn't figure out what in my head was rage and what was grief, but the resident's requests for diagnostic help had half of me thinking clinically. Like many other clinicians, once I am in clinical mode I can control negative emotions. I asked to review the medical chart, in order to make sense of how my grandfather had come to die without saying goodbye. The resident made me talk to his supervising physician, who allowed me to read the chart and did his best to explain what had happened.

It wasn't hard to piece together the story. Howard had a collection of blood about an inch in diameter at the base of his brain, in the wormy tangle of nerve tissue called the cerebellum. Blood in this location is notorious for causing a blockage of the flow of fluid out of the brain, leading to progressive sleepiness and then death from the effects of a swollen brain. The whole process takes about five days. Howard's final days could not have been more typical. Each morning the medical team documented that he was slightly sleepier than the day before, had some mild nausea, and was a little more forgetful. This process unfolded at its usual leisurely pace. I happened to come during the last half-hour of the disease course. While an inexperienced general medical doctor might not have known what to expect, the neurosurgeon certainly did. But the neurosurgeon saw Howard once, long enough to hear that Howard was DNR/DNI, and then disappeared. As best I could tell, the neurosurgeon never informed the medical team what to expect from the natural history of this bleeding without surgery. If the doctors had told anyone in our family that many patients in his situation would die comfortably over the course of several days, we could have all come to his deathbed. We could have honored Howard as he departed and heard his last words of wisdom before the swelling of his brain robbed him of consciousness. Instead we had an agitated flurry of activity and I—the grandson who had followed an intuition to come and visit and even so came twenty-four hours too late—was the only one even approximately on time to Granddad's death-bed. I wanted to shake the resident and his supervisor and tell them that DNI should mean, first and foremost, "Do Not Ignore."

The team had lost situational awareness by anchoring to the initial question—"will Howard undergo surgery?" Once that question was answered they forgot to follow it with, "what is likely to happen to Howard in the next few days if he refuses surgery?" Had they asked that second question, they would have realized that Howard had a brief window for wrapping up his life. The clinicians' failure to think clearly stole from Howard his chance for a good death.

My grandfather's example emphasizes the tendency of the current focus on procedures to distort clinicians' thinking. "What procedures did this patient refuse at some time in the past?" is the question that gets asked, not "What matters most to Howard and his family when his life is threatened?" or "How can we best support human flourishing at this phase of Howard's life?"

My experience with my grandfather's death early in my career was perhaps my first introduction to distractions from quality, human-centered care. Our family is only one of innumerable families harmed by an inhuman system. We need something better. We ought to demand something that honors us as human beings and prevents interference from predictable cognitive errors.

There is much at stake because as we will see in the next chapter, the ICU and the life-threatening illnesses treated there are soul-stretching and sometimes annihilating experiences.

Chapter 5

The Barbaric Life of
the Intensive Care Unit

She was slender but not yet wasting away, and she wore the head-dress of the chemotherapy patient with defiant pride. At seventy-nine, Joan anticipated that she would outlive her father, who had made it to ninety-nine.

Her cancer, small cell of the lung, is nearly always fatal, but it often gives people a brief holiday after the first round of chemotherapy. A sudden illness had interrupted Joan's holiday, though: She had what some call "chemo pneumonia." Many problems can cause the often fatal syndrome, and a sample drawn from the lung through a flexible scope passed through the mouth is usually necessary to identify the specific cause. As Joan's daughter reviewed the x-rays with me at the computer, Joan breathed quickly and uncomfortably from her hospital bed ten feet away. Sixty-five liters of pure oxygen blew toward her face every minute. As her daughter and I discussed the risks and benefits of bronchoscopy, Joan called out, "If that doctor is talking about death, you throw him right out of the room."

Joan repeated her mantra every time I entered the room that day. I didn't dare talk about the very real risk of death after such a stern warning. Joan was not delirious. She was a strong-willed, vivacious woman who had made clear that she did not want to talk about death with me, the intensive care unit (ICU) physician she had just met. So we made plans for full medical support.

The next morning Joan's condition had worsened, but her denial of death continued unchanged. It was time to intubate her or decide to allow a natural death. Then, unexpectedly, a cross-covering oncologist stopped by and spoke openly with Joan about the stark reality that her lung cancer would not respond to further chemotherapy. Hearing the news from him, Joan chose to make time to bid her family farewell and begin hospice. She died a day later. Straight talk from an oncologist was what it took for Joan to acknowledge her impending mortality and begin the process of saying goodbye. She almost lost the chance to bid farewell to her family; she almost became one of the many whose final moments are deformed or entirely erased by the ICU.

Despite recent improvements, the ICU remains a terrifying place. Loud alarm noises and occasional sobbing or calls of distress from neighboring rooms disrupt sleep continually, tubes get placed in every imaginable orifice, and the body begins to ache terribly due to immobility from days spent in bed. Communication is terrible as a rule, with long periods of waiting uncertainly for what is too often bad news.

Few places are less suited to rational decisions or emotional health than the ICU. For patients, the anxiety of illness is often accompanied by confusion as the brain stops functioning normally. Fear of death can keep clinicians and patients from discussing anything beyond the technical details of the ICU treatments, as I, to my discredit, had done with Joan. Physicians have trouble focusing on anything beyond the risky procedures and high-stakes diagnostic evaluations they perform when time is of the essence. It's no wonder that advance directives hope to avoid unwanted ICU admissions.

Medical professionals generally work in ICUs because they love the intensity of the job, the flow of adrenalin that comes with rushing to save a person's life. The clinicians' love of the hectic pace and the technical sophistication of life support procedures tend to draw attention away from what matters most to people. We who work in the ICU know that our treatments are sometimes barbaric, but we keep that knowledge at bay because we have seen the benefits those treatments can bring. This step can create a kind of fatalism about how stressful life support therapies and the surrounding ICU environment have to be. Some clinicians believe the status quo is just how things are: They're saving lives; they cannot also run a yoga studio or psychotherapist's office.

When you are a patient in the ICU, the deck is stacked against you. You feel terrible. If you weren't extremely sick, you wouldn't be in the

ICU in the first place. Many ICU treatments make speech and communication difficult if not impossible. You are frightened, often beyond words. You often do not understand what is happening, and your first impulse may be to hope that ignorance will, if just this once, really be bliss. You feel conflicted, uncertain how to receive or process the information presented to you. You are in unfamiliar territory, drowning in data but starved for useful information. Time is compressed—many decisions need to be made over the course of minutes or hours and do not allow for sustained deliberation. Even when you are conscious, you are in no condition to reason carefully or weigh risks and benefits. The alarms never stop chirping, chiming, or bellowing. Sometimes you're in the ICU for days, sometimes weeks or even months. You will likely have dramatic nightmares or hallucinations. Some of those false memories may haunt you for years afterward.

People are admitted to ICUs at many different phases of life. Some are perfectly healthy until a car accident or brain aneurysm brings them to death's door. Some have chronic illnesses like heart failure that flare up or make them so vulnerable that a minor illness like a bladder infection gets the best of them. And some come to die because until the ICU admission clinicians have failed to communicate well or everyone has been in denial about how sick they really were.

Beyond whatever medical condition brought them to the ICU in the first place, all patients and families admitted to the ICU with serious illness are at high risk for acute emotional and moral suffering, and, for some, a deformed death. Although each group of patients has very different needs, the current medical system treats them largely the same. A healthful, humane ICU will require close attention to the unique needs and concerns of patients and families.

The ICU is where the rubber hits the road in terms of advance directives and the stress of life-threatening illness. Because living wills function so poorly and the ICU generally emphasizes technology over humanity, families sometimes still allow unnecessarily brutal treatments when a loved one is in the ICU. Families intend well. They want more than anything for their loved one to survive.

In one painful afternoon about a decade ago I exhausted two hospitals' supplies of adrenalin in a desperate attempt to treat Bruce's overwhelming shock. He had already been mostly dead for two weeks when that final afternoon came. His three daughters stood by his bedside, screaming at me and threatening lawsuits if I let him die. Finally Bruce's heart stopped and there was not even anything unreasonable left to do. "Dad, the doctors killed you!" one daughter yelled, as the monitor announced that his heart rate was finally zero.

While extreme, versions of this scenario take place every week in ICUs across the United States. Discussions of episodes like this tend to focus on the financial cost of "futile" care, but weightier problems than finances are at stake. Because of our nation's relentless commitment to invasive, uncomfortable treatments, neither Bruce nor his daughters had been able to say goodbye or reflect on the meaning of his life before his final illness. He had been pinned to a hospital bed for months, comatose except for episodes of extreme pain, and then he was gone, in a storm of anger and recrimination. Bruce's daughters' rage seemed to express in part their regret that the medical system had stolen from them a farewell appropriate to their love for their father.

Bruce's story isn't typical of the contemporary ICU. But while extreme, it illuminates the general tensions that exist there, even if such an obvious human catastrophe is rare. More commonly, families adjust over time to the reality of a patient's final decline. But even if most families do not demand that we assault the dying the way we did Bruce, ICUs still stand in desperate need of reform.

Intensive care units are special places, the showrooms of what many call the "culture of rescue," wherein we prevent death, with great technological sophistication, at a given moment in time. Until recently, however, physicians and researchers did not look beyond that moment of crisis. We knew almost nothing about life after the ICU. Even today, most physicians don't know much about patient-relevant outcomes after critical illness. Yet life after the ICU is becoming more and more common. Whereas once 80 to 90 percent of very sick patients died despite intensive care, now about 80 percent survive. Living wills arose when most people died in ICUs, when we knew almost nothing about life in and after the ICU. Both of those facts have changed dramatically in the last twenty years. What happens in the ICU matters, a lot. Certain aspects of life in the ICU need to be called by name in order to see their influence on our thinking more clearly. Unnamed, they have a tendency to create persistent blind spots.

THE INTENSIVE CARE UNIT
IS A BRUTAL PLACE

I'm aware that my choice of words may be scandalous. But here I repeat my claim that much of what I do as an ICU physician is barbaric. Acute life support therapies and the ICU experience are often brutal. If someone performed these same acts on an enemy combatant, those procedures would constitute *torture*, inhuman and terrifying. This brutality is a key source of the moral distress clinicians experience.

I hope this kind of honest assessment will ultimately allow clinicians to see their professional lives in a new light. Of course, ICU clinicians perform their barbaric procedures because they want the patient to recover, and as a consequence their behaviors do *not* constitute torture. These brutish treatments are attempts to keep a body alive long enough that it can begin to heal from a physical crisis. But the procedures look enough like torture that they activate the parts of clinicians' souls that are justly horrified by physical cruelty. To deal with that horror, many clinicians push the pain away, which can lead to both pessimism, as we've seen, and fatalism.[1] That avoidant fatalism has, I believe, contributed to the brutality experienced in the ICU by separating clinicians from the human experience of patients.

There are reasons for some of the cruel aspects of life support therapy. The beds are lumpy and uncomfortable because they need to be easily sanitized between patients and need to contort into a hundred different shapes to allow clinicians to perform difficult procedures safely. The tubes we insert into patients' orifices (including the consummately private ones) usually enter the body with a clear therapeutic purpose. We humans did not evolve to live through the kinds of illnesses that we now survive with life support, and there's no reason to think that our bodies would have evolved to find life support comfortable.

No one sets out to be physically cruel to sick people when they design or use life support systems. The goal is to preserve life. But life support is still miserable and painful, even sometimes disfiguring. We as medical professionals make it through the day by knowing that even though we're doing something painful, we are doing it for a worthy cause. Not just a worthy cause in general terms (that is, after all, how interrogators justify actual torture), but a cause worthy to the individual undergoing that treatment. So we make an uneasy truce with the brutality of our therapies, and we hope that our patients recover.

When clinicians become pessimistic about the chance that a given patient will recover, they may find themselves suddenly without a hedge against the brutality. They lose the ability to explain what they're doing as anything but barbarism. I've mentioned that moral distress can cause undue pessimism or premature cessation of treatments. I have also witnessed a kind of fatalistic brutalism—things seems so bad that some minor brutality couldn't make things worse.

One simple example will stand in for many others. When patients appear to be unconscious, clinicians perform tests to determine the degree of unconsciousness. Sometimes new problems can arise in the brain, and if clinicians ignore the descent from moderate to severe coma, they may miss something important, like bleeding into the brain. So clinicians see whether they can rouse the patients from deep coma by shouting, pushing hard against the breastbone, squeezing the fingernails with a pen laid crosswise over the cuticle, or digging a finger into a ridge on the top of the eye socket, toward the middle, where a tiny nerve runs. The last two are extremely painful techniques that could be used in torture chambers. The idea behind them is that this pain will rouse even a very damaged brain without leaving any physical scar.

I've seen clinicians squeeze the fingernails of patients who respond to a loud voice. This is often just silly excess—if you respond to a loud voice, your brain is basically awake, no matter what you do when someone squeezes your finger. There are exceptions, such as needing to confirm that each individual limb can move, and there are probably advantages to knowing as much as possible about what's going on with a given patient. But we haven't studied this question well enough to know the best way to test brain function in patients who are unconscious in the ICU. How often do we need to test it? What will happen if we don't cause fingernail pain? What will happen if we do? We haven't asked those questions, so we go on inflicting deep pain at arbitrary intervals in people whose brains are already under siege.

The practice of inflicting pain for sometimes unnecessary neurological examinations is only the tip of the iceberg of things we do in the ICU that don't need to be done that way. But the practices persist in part because it's too distressing to think of the patient in the bed as a human being, besieged as we all are by the specter of death.

We live our lives specifically; that specificity is the fabric of our identity. Even the horrifying assault of life-threatening illness is something we experience individually. To avoid the generic and theoretical approach that bedevils advance directives, it's worth having concrete knowledge about what the ICU—a place of rapid, dramatic change and many threats to health and life—is actually like.

Patients in the ICU typically have experience with the ventilator, bed rest, catheters, and delirium. While other life support treatments exist, they are similar enough to others that I don't consider them separately here.[2]

The Experience of the Ventilator

Medicine has made dramatic advances since the Copenhagen polio epidemic that inaugurated the respiratory/medical ICU. Breathing tubes are now commonplace, and ventilators are small and sophisticated, some the size of a child's lunchbox. A small balloon inflates and holds the breathing tube in place within the windpipe, while preventing bacteria-laden secretions from falling down into the lungs (many modern tubes incorporate a suction system just above the balloon to keep that area clear and thereby decrease the risk of pneumonia).

Although many improvements have been put in place, most people find mechanical ventilation uncomfortable at first. For many people, it feels like a stranger has stuck a finger down their throat. Some people find the ventilator so unnerving that they require a medical coma to calm them, although such induced comas have been grossly overused. This isn't universally true; not everyone hates it. Particularly after they have been on the ventilator for a few days, some patients become reasonably comfortable. Many of them walk around the ICU on the ventilator.

I have patients who—under full support of the mechanical ventilator—text, tweet, and Facebook as efficiently as any distracted teen ignoring his parents.

Most patients on the ventilator have, however, a limited ability to communicate. Research is underway to understand whether some adaptive technologies could be harnessed to support better communication while on the ventilator—including virtual reality, eye-driven tablets, and robotic arms. None of these technologies has yet become mainstream.

Researchers have experimented with various ways of programming ventilators. Some ventilator modes do appear to be slightly more comfortable for patients, although research in actual patient comfort on the ventilator is in its infancy. The reality is that, as best as we can tell, the discomfort of the ventilator is mostly from the damn tube down the throat and the breathlessness that comes from the disease itself.

The biggest problem with the ventilator is that people whose lung disease or shock is grave enough to threaten their lives are often unable to survive long enough for the ventilator to become tolerable. They may move from uncomfortable confusion to death without ever communicating meaningfully with their families.

Immobilization

People in the ICU are often so sick that their bodies can barely move. Historically, clinicians' anxiety about patients' physical safety led to a regimen of strict bed rest. A mixture of sedating medications and physical restraints made this system work. When I was in training we used padded leather handcuffs. These days are long gone, but the inclination to restrain remains. The ties on wrists and occasionally torsos that clinicians use now aren't as barbaric as some of the restraints that were once employed—they are soft, foamy things nowadays—but they still tie the person to the bed.

A friend's elderly father, a devout Catholic, received his last rites in a hospital. He struggled against the wrist restraints to create the sign of the cross in response to the priest's gentle ministration. The restraints intended to keep him from dislodging any medical equipment obstructed his desperate hunger to participate in the healthful rituals of the deathbed. He died later that day. It never occurred to the nurses and doctors to release the restraints for this final interaction with his priest. My friend and his family still remember that angry straining for divine connection, stymied by medical handcuffs.

Some patients are like toddlers in a china shop, needing either constant attention or the restraints. Many in the ICU community think it would require a full-time person standing at the bedside twenty-four hours per day to keep such patients safe. Sometimes, family members are able to take shifts at the bedside to "reorient" the patient and keep her from harming herself accidentally. That's probably the best solution, but it's exhausting for family members. There are still rare patients who are so sick that when they awaken even a little bit their bodies fall apart—their oxygen levels drop through the floor and their heart comes under serious strain. Those patients may still need to be kept asleep and possibly restrained, but they are the decided minority.

It's easy to understand—and even, if we are fair, sympathize with—the nurses who use restraints on their patients. Unrestrained people on the mechanical ventilator do remove their breathing tubes sometimes, and an event like that can, rarely, be fatal. But the truth is that even restrained patients remove their breathing tubes sometimes and about half of patients who remove their breathing tubes on their own don't even need to have them reinserted. Clinicians joke nervously that the "patient knows best" when that happens, but there's some rueful truth lurking behind that phrase. Sometimes what everyone assumed was right turns out to have been wrong all along. Restraints in general may soon become the cruel relics of a bygone era.

In our ICUs at Intermountain Healthcare, we have observed that often people are less delirious and less anxious if we get them up out of bed and walk them around the ICU. The walking both gives them something to do with their restlessness and wears them out enough that they can fall asleep when they get back in bed. We have committed physical therapists who work together with nurses to march patients around the unit in promenades they call the "bag and drag" because oxygen is delivered by the therapist rhythmically squeezing a special bag attached to the breathing tube and the support lines and medications drag behind the patient as she makes her way around the ICU. Twenty years ago these patients would have been tied to a bed in a drug-induced coma.

We're not the only group doing this. The academic societies are rallying behind the concept, and many ICUs have caught the vision of patients awake and walking. We could all do better, though. In too many ICUs, being sick still means being drugged up and tied to a bed.[3]

Tubes and More Tubes

"Catheter" is the medical term for a flexible, hollow tube, something like a sterile drinking straw. Bodies under the assault of a life-threatening illness are unable to perform many key functions for themselves. These functions include elimination of waste and the circulation of blood and air in their respective bodily compartments. We use catheters for three main purposes: to drain fluids or wastes from the body, to instill medications or fluids into the body, and to make measurements inside the body.

The catheters we use to support failing hearts and treat shock are called "central venous catheters."[4] These flexible sterile tubes snake their way from the large jugular vein in the neck or the big vein under the collarbone to a spot just before the blood enters the heart. An older model that we don't use much anymore went all the way through the heart up into the arteries inside the lungs. With support catheters in place, we can infuse adrenalin and other life-sustaining medications. While they're sometimes uncomfortable to insert—patients often feel claustrophobic under the sterile drape used to prevent bacterial contamination of the bloodstream—most patients aren't bothered much by the catheters.

Even when they're awake, ICU patients are commonly too weak to manage their own bowel and bladder functions. Catheters have tiny balloons near their tips that hold them inside the bladder or the rectum and allow evacuation of waste. These catheters prevent wet and soiled beds and probably decrease the chance of bedsores, but they are prone to infection because they provide a pathway from the outside world of germs to the normally sterile inside of the body.

Medical professionals tend to think of these catheters as innocuous, but that is only because most have not had one placed in themselves. When I fractured my ankle in a fall in the White Mountains of New

Hampshire, I had to crawl off a mountain with a broken leg for twelve hours and then drive back to the hospital in Boston to have surgery. I have two main memories of the discomfort associated with the fractured leg: the moment when my spinal anesthetic wore off, and the pain from the catheter placed into my bladder in order to drain urine during surgery. The instant the pain had eased some in my leg, I felt like I was being stabbed in my nether parts. The pain was sharp enough that I started rifling through the drawers of the cabinet next to my bed looking for a syringe so that I could remove the catheter myself. The nurse relented and removed the catheter.

My mind was clear, so I experienced only the physical discomfort of the bladder catheter. Critically ill patients are often not so fortunate: Some of them remember the catheter as a sexual assault. The majority don't report the delusion, but it's common for female patients to have memories of rape from urinary bladder catheters. While healthcare workers get harangued constantly about overuse of those catheters by the regulators because of the risk of bladder infection, I've started to wonder whether, in the ICU, the risk of delusions of rape should be a more important reason to avoid the catheters whenever possible. Unfortunately, there isn't yet a reliable way to avoid these catheters for the sickest patients.

One poor woman with terrible lung injury still haunts me. Her delusional memories of the bladder catheter were particularly intense and long-lived. The resident physician I was supervising at the time was muscular and quiet, a steely alpha male, and the patient had a history of relationships with similar men. When she awoke from the medical coma we'd been forced to use to keep oxygen circulating through her lungs, her memory was not of rape but of consensual intercourse. The resident, in her memory, had impregnated her and promised to marry her. We finally had to reassign the poor resident because she either treated him as her fiancé with ostentatious displays of affection or screamed at him for trying to break the betrothal. I'm embarrassed to admit that it didn't occur to us at the time to connect her with a psychiatrist or grief counselor to process these delusions and their aftermath, as we now know to do. Mostly we laughed sheepishly at how strange and regrettable the situation was. Similarly terrible false memories may be associated with

equivalent catheters sometimes used to manage diarrhea in unconscious patients.[5]

THE BRAIN UNDER SIEGE

Intensive care unit treatments are all bad enough, as they go, but problems with patients' brains are especially troublesome. Troubles with the
brain shape the experience of everything in the ICU, with lasting conse-
quences. The brain is under assault during most life-threatening illness.
There are several words to describe this state—delirium, encephalopathy, brain injury—but they all refer to altered states of consciousness
related to brain dysfunction. It's a lot like being drunk: spooky, frightened, frantic drunk. An inflamed brain works about as well as a wet computer. In the last twenty years, with particular contributions made by
groups at Vanderbilt University and Intermountain Healthcare, we've
come to understand a lot more about the brain during and after the ICU.

The best-studied of the physical brain syndromes is called sepsis-
associated encephalopathy. In sepsis, the whole body is bathed in chemical hormones that cause blood vessels to leak and tissues to swell. The
lungs fill with fluid, the liver clogs with bile, the kidneys stop making
urine, and the limbs swell as if they've all been sprained. The inflammation affects the brain as much as the rest of the body. While researchers
have begun to understand more about the chemical processes involved,
our insight into the phenomenon is mostly limited to the suggestion that
some of the medications we've used as sedatives are probably contributing to the problem.[6]

The swollen brain reverts to a very simplistic way of processing
information and creating memories. In this state, even the nonrational-
ity of System 1 is a pipe dream. Partial, damaged memories can create
echoes far into the future.

The rape delusions associated with bladder catheters are haunt-
ing enough, but they don't exhaust the list of terrible memories people
often acquire in the ICU. Most of these frightening delusions relate to
imprisonment, capture, or torture. Some feature aliens or homicidal
doctors and nurses. More than a few incorporate the famous Capgras

delusion, in which the important people in a person's life are replaced by evil duplicates. These interpretations likely derive from the intense, paranoid attention that comes with high stress coupled with acute pain. The distressed brain tries to weave a meaningful narrative to explain why familiar faces (or people in professional gear and lab coats) are poking and prodding you as you are tied to a bed. Some delusions are more benign, perhaps tied to the soft and undulating hospital beds: British researchers report delusions about going on cruises. (I haven't encountered anyone with that delusion; there may be cultural differences at play here, perhaps driven by Europeans' love of long vacations.)[7] While delusions run the gamut, some are frankly horrifying.

Some delusional memories are less traumatic and more just plain weird. Emily was a strong, athletic woman, suddenly struck by Legionnaires' disease, an uncommon and sometimes devastating cause of pneumonia. Very low oxygen levels kept her in the ICU for a couple extra days after she was breathing on her own, but she was clearly coming back to herself. She and I had bonded for three days after she got off the ventilator, telling jokes and getting to know each other a little. When I visited her in the rehabilitation facility two weeks later, she had no memory of me at all. I asked her what memories she had before her return to memorable consciousness a day or two after she arrived at the rehabilitation center. She had two memories, one vague and one extremely distinct.

The vague memory is one I've heard from other people over the years: bats. I suspect it has to do with the endless whistling noises of the ventilator and all the other rustling around the hospital bed. The patients' memories are rarely, in my experience, terribly clear. There's commonly a sense of small things moving about together in an ominous way—sometimes it's bats, sometimes mice. Alcoholics classically hallucinate about ants crawling under their skin; the brains of ICU patients have their own methods for creating delusional narratives to explain vexing physical sensations during a period of altered consciousness. Whatever the facts, Emily remembered lying in bed semiconscious, covered in bats that flapped their wings in her face endlessly. Such are the plots for low-budget horror movies, not what we would wish for when we are sick.

Emily's second delusional memory was much more distinct, and it has stayed with me for years. She was a stuffed grizzly bear in a museum in Yellowstone. She watched from behind thick glass as the world streamed past her, but she was a dry-embalmed bear locked in a display case. Even without being a Freudian, it seems pretty clear that Emily was trying to make sense of the deep depersonalization of lying half awake tied to an ICU bed. In my experience most of the delusions have some tie to real experience, however tenuous.

One older woman from rural Idaho had a perfectly clear memory of walking down a country lane with russet potatoes glowering at her like the stone heads of Easter Island. She wasn't sure what the potatoes were trying to say—the sounds emanating from them were indistinct, like the buzzing that other patients experience as bats—but she knew they meant trouble.

A blessed few ICU survivors have memories that sustain them, grand visions of God or afterlife. But those types of memories, termed "near death experiences" by some, are vanishingly rare in my experience. Occasionally I hear reports of ghostly visits—especially from deceased family members—a story as old as recorded human history. But the vast majority of people who move through an ICU during a life-threatening illness do not remember anything so reassuring or delightful as a near-death experience. For the overwhelming majority of people, actual near-death experiences—life in that state of suspended animation that hovers between life and death—are painful, demoralizing, and disorienting.[8]

It's anyone's best guess why precisely these memories arise. Some of it is clearly the medications clinicians use to help patients stay calm. All of the current medicines disrupt perception and memory at the same time that they help people be quieter and more comfortable on the ventilator. We know from ambulatory surgery and minor procedures that a certain number of people who get the same medications will sometimes have funny dreams or misperceptions. But it's not just the medications creating delusions in the ICU. There's something else going on.

Delusions in the ICU probably share some mechanisms with dreams. People tend to hallucinate about things that worry them, much as they might have recurring dreams. A recent fire in the neighborhood may create dreams about burning or a particular delusion in the ICU about one's home burning to the ground.[9] A study in Britain found that ICU hallucinations might incorporate details from television news stories.[10] In my own experience with patients, hallucinations commonly incorporate objects from the environment, like the alarm clock that becomes an air raid siren or the droning of alarms that become bats. Reports from Britain suggest that almost nine out of ten patients admitted to the ICU for more than three days have delusional memories.[11] That staggeringly high number is no surprise: Patients are half-asleep, their brains bathed in the chemical hormones of the stress response smothered in tranquilizers, and then they are asked to interpret unfamiliar, uncomfortable stimuli.

Given that there are so many terrible experiences at play and so much misgiving about how to proceed or when to stop, one would think that we in the medical system would have developed techniques to ease the burdens of brain dysfunction. Ways to guide people through the experiences that confront them in the ICU. But the truth is that we are in the Stone Age when it comes to communication and human support in the ICU. That fact is the main reason I have written this book.

I include a discussion of the failure of communication here because I strongly believe that excellent communication is a procedure as significant as any that we perform in the ICU. It is desperately, morally wrong that we don't pay much attention to it in our training or in our efforts to measure and improve the quality of medicine.

POOR COMMUNICATION IS COMMON IN THE INTENSIVE CARE UNIT

Copious research shows that, whatever we think of ourselves, ICU clinicians, like most people, are on average not great communicators. Related research shows that this poor communication harms patients and families: They make worse decisions and suffer as a result. A few communication training programs have surfaced, mostly for cancer clinicians.[12] These programs get at the basics: You should listen, make sure people understand, provide context, validate people's emotions, and make sure you have communicated accurately. It's the kind of simple stuff that people with social skills know automatically and that you could get from a decent community college adult education class in "Communication." But high-quality communication is rare enough in ICU medicine that you'd think it was an unsolved puzzle of quantum physics.

Just because it's inexcusable doesn't mean the communication failures aren't understandable. Schedules are crowded, people are tired, events happen unexpectedly, and the stakes are high. The sad reality is that communication in the ICU has been a disaster for a very long time. But it doesn't have to be that way. Effective communication requires constant vigilance and attention to the needs and perspectives of the patient and family. I still remember my failure with Susan and her family.

Susan's family told me you'd never meet a more cheerful person. She was a top-notch aunt who never refused an opportunity to make a child's day brighter. On Monday, she got a bit of a sore throat and a mild fever with chills. She toughed out this "flu" for a couple of days and then went to an Instacare for a Strep test. The Strep test was negative, and the doctor advised rest and plenty of fluids. She took that advice, her four-year-old nephew, Soren, trucking back and forth to the kitchen to bring her jelly beans and cans of lemon-lime soda. Then Susan's breathing started to feel labored, and she worried that she had come down with a full-blown pneumonia, so her brother Royal bundled her up and took her to the hospital on Thursday. She started on the regular hospital floor, with the presumption that she had a viral pneumonia because her liver was showing some signs of irritation and her chest x-ray demonstrated subtle shadows. By Friday afternoon, Susan's body had fallen apart completely, every organ in disarray.

We'd had a tricky and memorable case a few years prior in which we had diagnosed the hemophagocytosis ("eating the blood") syndrome, a rare disorder in adults with which our ICU has gained unfortunate experience.[13] This rare and devastating disease of cells called macrophages is almost always fatal by the time a person reaches the ICU, so diagnosing it is more about naming the cause of death than having a chance for survival. It's almost like a cancer that unfolds in five days instead of five months as these macrophages eat the entire body, tissue by tissue. The most striking image from bone marrow biopsy is of the macrophages eating the oxygen-carrying red blood cells, which is where the syndrome gets its name. It's not a disease to wish on anybody, not even your worst enemy.

Susan looked for all the world like she had the hemophagocytosis syndrome, and we immediately began a combination of diagnostic tests and harsh chemotherapy for the disease. I spent the next eighteen hours struggling to keep Susan alive. A case like hers could keep the senior physician awake all night even if she were the only patient in the ICU. Every twenty minutes there was a new crisis that required a rapid response: lungs, heart, kidneys, clotting factors in her blood were all depleted. She was so sick I didn't dare leave her side, even for an hour. By the end of that marathon of intensive care, we had done everything we could, but her heart had stopped twice and was headed for its third stoppage. I checked her eyes quickly as I made my way through my checklist of possible complications and next steps.

Sometimes the eyes hold the secret to the status of the brain. Her saucer-sized pupils rebuked me by failing to constrict when I shined a light directly into her eyes. Susan died a few minutes later when her heart stopped, and no amount of energetic banging on her chest was able to restore her to life.

I hadn't opened Susan's eyes in the last hour of her life. I was focused on keeping her heart beating and generating a blood pressure compatible with life. I always regret missing something, even if it would not have changed the ultimate outcome. It's part of the obsession that drives most clinicians. We can't stand to be blindsided by a diagnosis.

Dilated pupils that don't respond to light can be a sign of brain death, especially as the result of significant bleeding into the brain. Or dilated pupils can just mean the patient received large doses of adrenalin. We had chosen not to treat her thin blood because giving clotting proteins doesn't make a difference when there is no obvious bleeding. As I mourned her death, I worried that Susan had died of preventable bleeding into the brain.

There's a microscope you carry in your back pocket as a physician. You whip it out to inspect your actions when the slightest thing goes wrong. You sometimes spend hours reviewing a single action you took or decided not to take. Like most physicians I know, I am my own harshest critic. Every act of criticism carries with it the possibility that I failed to save someone through my carelessness or lack of skill. This self-criticism is not my favorite part of my job. But I think it's necessary, however painful.

Because we wanted to be absolutely certain about the diagnosis, I recommended an autopsy, and Susan's family agreed. We made plans that I would follow up with her brother Royal once I had the results, because the rest of Susan's family wanted to be sure they understood precisely what had happened. I had been open with them about the possibility that she had suffered bleeding into the brain that had contributed to her death. I was confident about hemophagocytosis but worried about her brain.

I joined the pathologist for the autopsy the next morning. While autopsies remain a bizarre and uncomfortable ritual no matter how many of them I've seen, Susan's was a relief to me. Not that the fact of an autopsy is ever good news; it is, after all, a marker of a patient's death that left unanswered questions. But if an autopsy has to happen, the physician most wants to hear that he or she made the correct diagnosis and chose properly at each point along the way. The autopsy confirmed the hemophagocytosis syndrome, and the brain—while swollen and damaged just like the rest of the body by the malignant macrophages—was free of bleeding.

When I spoke with Royal later that day I emphasized the fact that the autopsy did not show the brain damage I had feared it might. My relief at having made the right call led me to focus on that finding early in our conversation. Royal began a verbal dance full of pauses in which he tried to decide what to tell the rest of his family. It took me a minute to catch on, but Royal soon changed my entire understanding of the autopsy.

Susan's family had started to make peace with her death by focusing on the possibility that she had suffered irreparable brain damage before the end. Compared with permanent brain damage, death became the lesser of two evils. In the early phase of their grieving, that was what they had held onto, the likelihood that she had bled into her brain and that consciousness had permanently fled before her heart stopped beating.

Our different needs for a meaningful story about Susan's autopsy were at cross-purposes. I needed to believe that I had not missed a serious cause of bleeding into the brain, and her family needed to believe that her death was a release from a body that had lost its personhood. I could hear the strain associated with navigating that tension in Royal's voice. I immediately adjusted my approach and began to describe the ways hemophagocytosis had ravaged her brain. Even without any bleeding, Susan had experienced serious brain damage. By the end of our rebooted conversation, Royal seemed more at peace, and I was both embarrassed and grateful.

Both ways of understanding the autopsy were true to the facts, but only one was actually of service to Susan's grieving family. In retrospect I should have listened before speaking. I could have started by asking, "Autopsies often include lots of different pieces of information that may be helpful or may be irrelevant. Can you tell me how you've been thinking about her death and what information the autopsy might provide in helping you understand her death better?" I don't think people would feel that they were being set up if the doctor started a conversation with a clarifying question. Since my mishap with Royal I've been trying to ask more questions before I start talking. This process of becoming attuned to the needs and perspectives of patients and families can take many forms. Communication isn't always limited to straightforward conversations.

WE DON'T ALWAYS KNOW WHAT WE WANT

In order to survive, many clinicians have made themselves relatively inaccessible to their patients. Coupled with deep reservations about getting tangled in the worldviews of strangers, we are sometimes silent or obtuse when we could say just the right words in great service to our patients. Just as some diseases require intense focus and experience to understand how they unfold, so do some individuals' values and priorities require special attention. A superficial view can lead clinicians and others to misinterpret what people want. It takes time and training to understand how to interpret heart sounds through a stethoscope, and it takes substantial attention to understand what patients say in a way that is consistent with their deeply held goals and aspirations.

In the ICU, as in so much of life, people don't always manage to say at first what it is they are trying to say. Communication requires finesse, careful attention, and ongoing negotiation.

Sometimes intuition is required.

In my first year out of medical school I took care of Mrs. Nadall on the cancer ward. She was on hospice, a decision she made carefully and in consultation with her family and physicians, for advanced pancreatic cancer that hadn't responded to chemotherapy, but she landed in the hospital because her family was struggling to control her pain. The nurses were doing a reasonable job with pain management, but she was clearly dying, with ever-lower oxygen levels in her blood.

She and her son called me to the room, frantic, shortly before she died. "Hallelujah," she exclaimed. "An angel of the Lord has told me that I will live, and I must go on the respirator."

I was initially at a loss, wanting to honor her wishes but uncertain what those wishes actually were. In a burst of inspiration I saw her not as a wavering, hallucinating patient, but as a frightened woman requesting reassurance in the face of death. Without thinking, I asked her slowly, "Are you ready to be with Jesus?" Not sure where those words came from—I am not an evangelical Protestant, and this question was not in the language of my faith—I followed the inexplicable force of intuition and asked again quietly. "Are you ready to be with Jesus?" "Yes," she answered with visible clarity and renewed vigor. She was not addressing me, though; she was speaking to her son, to a hoped-for afterlife, to the God whom she saw in the prospect of death without a ventilator. "Yes, I am ready to meet the Lord." I felt the fearful energy of her son at my side, but hoped he would find in her faith the confidence that the respirator would only postpone a glorious meeting with God. She requested morphine for her breathlessness, which I prescribed. She died about an hour later, with peaceful clarity.

I am still not entirely sure what happened that night with Mrs. Nadall, but that's not for a lack of trying. I've been pondering the encounter for years. When I poll audiences during ethics lectures, I am struck by how naturally they condemn my actions that night. When

I pose the question, listeners almost uniformly recommend intubation. She requested the respirator, they tell me, and I should have complied with her request without question. I had blocked her self-determination. Their certainty generally dissolves when we explore the case more carefully. As I have considered Mrs. Nadall's situation over the years, four possible explanations predominate:

1. Mrs. Nadall was afraid, seeking reassurance in the face of her imminent decease;
2. She was delirious from low oxygen levels in her blood;
3. An angel had actually come into her room and instructed her to request intubation; or
4. She had authentically changed her mind and did in fact want to spend her last few days unable to communicate on a ventilator.

If she was frightened, my inserting a plastic breathing tube through her mouth into her windpipe would have been an assault, an abdication of my duty to comfort a woman in great distress. If she was hallucinating, I would be overriding explicit instructions she gave just days before when she was of sound mind, in full awareness of the current arc of her illness. There is of course the question of an actual supernatural visitor, a possibility I feel ill-suited to assess. In retrospect I think I believed that if she had actually changed her mind for some reason, angelic or otherwise, Mrs. Nadall would have asked again to be intubated. Had I responded in a strictly legalistic way, I would have either brutalized her last days by attaching her to a mechanical ventilator or turned a deaf ear to her plea for reassurance and human presence as she was departing life. Neither would have honored her as a person. I believe that the most likely explanation is that she wasn't making a technical claim in favor of mechanical ventilation at the end of life, she wanted comfort and reassurance as she stared into the void. Using language that was specific to her personality, I was able to provide that comfort.

Failures of communication and understanding can contribute to a serious problem in the contemporary ICU.

DEFORMING DEATH IN THE RUSH
TO RESCUE

The majority of ICU patients survive. The work clinicians do matters. Many of us repeat this mantra to ourselves to keep going on particularly difficult days or nights. But it's also true that somewhere between 10 and 20 percent of our patients will die. And negotiating the transition from expecting survival to expecting death is difficult. America manages it poorly in the ICU and elsewhere, and living wills don't seem to have helped. I've emphasized risks of stopping too early and thereby failing to honor the actual values and priorities of patients. But the risk on the other side is also serious.

Clinicians move quickly in the ICU; sometimes it seems like there is no speed between 0 and 120 miles per hour. That rush can incur substantial risks. Without careful attention, clinicians may steal from people the chance to complete their lives. We can also get blinders on for philosophical reasons: We sometimes deal with the burden of agency by denying death entirely. Daniel Callahan, one of the founders of American bioethics, has written eloquently about the risk of deforming death. For Callahan, physicians always want to try one more thing, address one more failing organ. In what he calls "technological brinksmanship," Callahan argues that physicians see patients as a collection of ailments, each one of which has a possible treatment. "Kidneys don't work, let's dialyze. Lungs are shot, let's ventilate." The focus on ailments and solutions tends to draw attention away from the whole person.[14]

I'm not sure that Callahan has entirely understood the dynamics of contemporary intensive care, but he is absolutely right about the risk of deforming death. Clinicians can get so wrapped up in the procedural drama at hand that they forget the human drama that moves alongside it. They can, inadvertently, steal from people opportunities to wrap up their lives and say goodbye. (Notice that living wills fall prey to the same error by focusing on lists of procedures rather than the individual's phase of life and the tasks appropriate to it.)

Michael was thirty-six years old when I met him. He came to an ER as a mystery, complaining of nerve pain in his hands and feet and exhibiting too little clotting protein in his blood. His breathing grew more labored by the hour. The ER doctor wondered whether his immune system was chewing up all of Michael's blood clotting cells and sent him to me in hopes of making a firm diagnosis. Michael arrived in the ICU on the verge of death. His blood pressure was terribly low, and he was breathing as fast as a sprinter at the end of a 100-meter race. I responded instinctively to the crisis. I explained to him that we would need to support his breathing and blood pressure and attach him to our various life support systems immediately. Michael was frightened but mostly seemed glad at the possibility of relief from the breathlessness.

Michael's wife Nancy was in the waiting room, and I asked the resident to tell her that we were proceeding with life support procedures without delay. We did so quickly. Right before we intubated him, Michael was still awake—frightened, and not at his best, but awake and conversant. After intubation, he was deeply unconscious. Nancy saw him shortly thereafter in a coma, attached to the ventilator. Michael died twelve hours later. As he was dying, we received the results from a blood culture that confirmed an initial suspicion that he had extremely severe infection. It was a garden-variety Strep infection, the kind that causes pneumonia, and he had come to the hospital late in the course of an overwhelming case. When the antibiotics hit his bloodstream in the ER, the Strep bacteria died in droves. Michael's immune system responded to these dead bacteria by kicking into overdrive. He died of what is called fulminant (from the Latin word for a lightning strike) sepsis.

As I watched Nancy, her body convulsing in sobs, I did not regret the quality of our medical care. We'd done everything we could think of to save Michael, even considered experimental therapies. But I regretted deeply that Nancy had never been able to say goodbye to her conscious husband or even to tell him she loved him and wished him the best. I knew at the time that I intubated Michael that he had a high risk of not surviving his stay in the ICU. I was fully committed to keeping those chances as high as possible. But I could have encouraged Nancy's presence as we carried Michael onto life support and beyond the capacity to communicate. Michael's and similar cases have persuaded me of the risks of stealing from people moments of tender clarity with their loved ones, even when aggressive treatment is the right thing to do.

Clinicians commit to a plan of care and execute that plan proficiently and expeditiously. We clinicians consistently fail to think through the human implications of our medical decisions. Contrary to Callahan's description, the problem is not that clinicians keep exploring treatment options. Patients are generally grateful when physicians are willing to explore every opportunity to help. The problem is that clinicians are not simultaneously weighing the risks and benefits of their decisions in terms of the human wounds they may inflict, their relevance to a given patient's phase of life, or the opportunities they may steal from patients. Clinicians routinely fail to explore how to "hope for the best but prepare for the worst," to give a best effort to get someone through a life-threatening illness but still plan ways not to steal from them the time they need to connect with the people they care about or to make some conclusion to their lives. This effort requires acknowledging openly the specter of that death, but such acknowledgment can be healthful. I explore some ways to address these problems in chapter 8.

I'm acutely aware of the incredible good done in ICUs all across the world, but the ICU remains a horrifying place. It's terrible both because of the diseases that require intensive care and because it imposes sometimes appalling burdens on both patients and clinicians. The current structure of ICUs can be ghastly for everyone involved. It often leaves patients drugged up and traumatized, their families demoralized, and the physicians morally distressed.

I'm aware that even though I love my clinical work, I've painted a stark picture of the ICU and the work I do as a clinician. We are at a point where the status quo must not persist. The obstacles are immense, but the situation is not hopeless. We as a medical community and a broader society need to understand what's painful about intensive care and what assistance people need as they make their way through life-threatening illness. We need to understand better how to tailor our approach to the specific person in the ICU bed. With those pieces in place, we can start to understand clearly what's wrong and what we need to do to fix intensive care. Intensive care units can remain technically proficient while becoming places for human healing. There is one more piece of the puzzle to explore here—what happens to people after they "graduate" from the ICU.

Chapter 6

Life after the Intensive Care Unit

Rich, barely fifty, walks with a walker.[1] His toes catch on the ground if he tries to rush, so he shuffles too slowly to wave the Nepalese prayer flags he has tied to the crossbeam of his walker. During the day he breathes a liter per minute of inhaled oxygen through a tube draped like a plastic moustache across his upper lip. He needs triple that dosage at night. He is finally starting to sleep through the night again, after several months of sleeping no more than three hours at a time. On better days, he jokes with his wife, Jessica, that he's been "born again": At age fifty he is living through a second infancy. "I'm learning to walk and eat and breathe, all over again. I just barely figured out how to wipe my own ass. I don't think this is what the Bible people mean when they talk about how great it is to be born again." On his off days, he's withdrawn, moody, and even bitter, a fact he's not proud of. He and Jessica fight sometimes, for no good reason. Certain sounds and smells trigger horrifying memories of his weeks in the ICU. These mostly delusional memories of his illness and hospitalization shake him to the core. The strongest memory he carries is of being tied to a bed and water-boarded to reveal America's nuclear secrets. He's more emotional and more spiritual than he was before, a fact he considers a silver lining in the dark cloud of his illness.

Four months after getting home, he is far from returning to work as a tax accountant. He wishes more than anything that he could get back to work. Sometimes he retrieves old annual reports and tries to remember what life was like when he wrote them, but he finds it difficult to keep more than one thing in his mind at a time and instead gets lost in the numbers like a child wandering in an unfamiliar forest. He's able to recognize a few of the trees but unable to visualize a path out of the woods.

Rich's saga started with a gallstone that got stuck in the bile duct and caused terrible inflammation of the pancreas, a condition called "gallstone pancreatitis." It is staggering to think that one little ball of hardened cholesterol smaller than the tip of a pinkie finger could cause an entire body to collapse. But it can: I've seen it many times. The gallstone blocks the duct that the pancreas shares with the liver, and the digestive juices of the pancreas go berserk. Like a laboratory technician spilling acid on his skin or a farmer inhaling pesticide, the pancreas's digestive chemicals wreak utter havoc. I've seen gallstone pancreatitis kill people outright in three miserable days, and I've seen people survive by the skin of their teeth.

Rich is one of our success stories. He was in our ICU for nine weeks. For the first three weeks it wasn't clear whether he would live or die. His lungs were so full of fluid we could barely persuade the ventilator to circulate oxygen through them; his blood pressure was so low that we had four different adrenalin infusions running. We had to dialyze him continuously to keep the acid levels in his blood out of the danger zone. His status changed hour by hour.

Finally Rich entered the state called "chronic critical illness." The definitions vary somewhat from study to study, but in general you have to be dependent on the ventilator or in the ICU for three or four weeks to qualify as chronically critically ill. A small but significant minority of patients move from their acute illness to this chronic state.[2]

Chronic critical illness, the fate of about 100,000 Americans at any given time, is something of a purgatory, although the metaphor isn't a perfect fit. In Catholic Purgatory you're in the state of purifying misery for a long enough time that you're finally righteous enough to make it into heaven. Purgatory is like an industrial washing machine—long, hot, and painful, but you ultimately come out clean. Traditionally some people may be caught in Catholic Purgatory for seemingly forever, but people don't sink from that purgatory into hell. For chronic critical illness, though, people can drop from purgatory straight to hell. A little over a third of patients with chronic critical illness do not survive their first year. For the two-thirds who do survive, the state can seem to extend forever. If they're lucky, the suffering counts as some sort of purification before they recover; if they're not lucky, they just suffered before they died.

Rich spent four months in a long-term acute care hospital (LTACH). These facilities, a cross between a hospital and a nursing home, have sprung up as more people are surviving long enough in the ICU to develop chronic critical illness. When they are pessimistic about the outcomes, physicians sometimes call LTACHs or similar facilities "vent farms," the agricultural allusion a disparaging reference to "vegetables." Physicians use the term to separate themselves from the distress of caring for patients who remain profoundly dependent after an ICU stay.

The LTACHs can be difficult places to work. They feel separated from the rest of medicine, there are fewer resources than in the acute care hospitals, and the patients and families are often traumatized by a surgery gone bad or a protracted ICU stay. The work is simultaneously demanding and discouraging. The families have often suffered from poor communication while in the original hospital and may have substantial misgivings about their new doctors, nurses, and therapists. The lucky LTACH patients graduate to a rehabilitation facility and then ultimately get to go home. The unlucky either die in the LTACH or transition to a permanent residence in a skilled nursing facility.

Rich was one of the lucky. He spent four weeks in rehabilitation until he finally reached the point that his doctor thought—with incredible support from Jessica—that he could make it at home. And he is making it. Slowly, tentatively, over months rather than days or weeks, Rich is making it.

The miracles of contemporary life support technology restore life where death was once imminent. These victories deserve our profound respect. These medical successes have brought with them a whole group of people now living on the other side of death. This is uncharted territory for our species: Our bodies didn't evolve to survive such injuries. In the words of one prominent researcher, ICU survivorship is the defining problem for the critical care community in the twenty-first century.[3]

The work we do as ICU clinicians has been designed to get people out of the ICU alive. That has been the focus since intensive care first developed fifty years ago. Only very recently has the ICU community begun to acknowledge what life looks like for patients after the ICU. Sometimes our patients and their families are as shell-shocked after ICU discharge as military combat veterans. Often they struggle with new physical and mental disabilities. Patients awaken with a body and mind that don't work as well as they once did but little or no memory of how they ended up there. Families—whether through the horrors of bereavement or the depleting care of a newly dependent loved one—experience their own afflictions as a result of the ICU experience.

Some of the emotional stress after an ICU stay is unavoidable, but much of the psychological suffering comes because the medical system adds insult to injury through failures to acknowledge and support the human needs of patients and their families. To date, society has mostly been satisfied counting bodies, dollars, and living wills rather than attending to the human beings that pass through the ICU. "Choose your bed," the system appears to say, "and then lie in it." But we shouldn't be asking people which medical procedures from our macabre menu they chose in a hypothetical thought experiment. Instead, we should work to transform the ICU to make it more responsive to people's actual needs, values, and aspirations while improving patient-centered outcomes.

Things are slowly starting to change. Physicians now have reliable information about what life looks like after the ICU; when living wills came into vogue, no one knew much about life after an ICU admission. These new insights—and the possibility of effective treatments and prevention—have come through the strivings of a group of thoughtful researchers who were willing to swim upstream for years, in order to better understand and support ICU survivors. They came to appreciate a wide array of important health problems that ICU survivors confront.

The creation of large and growing groups of ICU survivors is a promissory note. Clinicians promise that the care they provided in the ICU was a blessing rather than a curse. And the entire medical system owes on that promise. It's not enough to say, "You chose intensive care, so make peace with where it got you." We need to make life better for those who survived. That work is just beginning.

A FEW VISIONARY RESEARCHERS

The world of intensive care research has always been a complicated one. Medical care has tended to be organized around organ systems—a reflex of the reductionist turn in Western medicine in the early twentieth century. Intensive care arose within the specialist-dominated hospital and aimed to take on the problems of multiple organ systems at once. Intensive care wasn't one specialty, it was charged with handling the most frightening clinical problems of all the specialties.

Because critical care physicians took care of many different organ systems at once, rather than any single organ by itself, intensive care didn't fit into the traditional organ-based structure of the National Institutes of Health (NIH). But the NIH was the source of funding and legitimacy for medical research; without attention from the NIH, nothing was likely to happen. As the medical research community increasingly chased genes, proteins, and molecular pathways, it tended to ignore what it was like to be a human being confronted by illness. The laser-sharp focus on molecular medicine and the latest pharmaceutical therapeutics meant that research into the human side of life-threatening illness received short shrift.

Another simple structural issue made it difficult for ICU outcomes research to flourish. The divide between physicians and nurses often separates the worlds of biomedical science and human healing. Physician researchers were responsible for cold, hard facts about basic biology. They were preventing death after life-threatening illness, so let the cards fall where they may. Nurses were responsible for "soft" topics like communication or treating patients as persons. They were not to get in physicians' way.

But a few people resisted the consensus, founding what has become the thriving field of ICU outcomes research. They have made substantial scientific and clinical advances. Four researchers in particular have been the unsung heroes of people with life-threatening illness. Their efforts have pointed out several areas that matter and have given a name to a syndrome, the Post Intensive Care Syndrome (PICS), that organizes our thinking clinically and scientifically.

In Liverpool, lore has it that a physician named Eric Sherwood-Jones started the field of ICU outcomes research at Whiston Hospital in the 1960s. According to memories of those who followed him, Dr. Sherwood-Jones spent careful time seeing his ICU patients in his outpatient clinic after their discharge. By the time he retired in the 1980s, he had created a local tradition of ICU follow-up that began to support a research enterprise. Christina Jones, a nurse-psychotherapist, in collaboration with one of Sherwood-Jones's physician successors in Liverpool, added rigor to the study of the rehabilitation needs of ICU survivors.

The British are less prone to use intensive care than Americans are, but they provide top-notch care to the people who do end up in the ICU. Jones wrote her doctoral dissertation, Rehabilitation After Critical Illness, at the University of Liverpool. She developed a textbook and a rehabilitation manual for patients with advice, guidance, and signposts, including frank discussions about resuming sexual activity, how to pace one's breathing, how to walk safely when one's balance is off, and how to strengthen one's legs. The rehabilitation manual is definitely British—proposed markers of physical recovery include "ball room dancing" and "potter[ing] around the garden"—and it's not clear how well the text itself would work in the United States, where both general and medical culture differ from the UK. Still, Jones's careful studies suggest that the manual helps patients navigate the world after the ICU. In her randomized study of over one hundred patients, people who used the manual achieved better ultimate physical function than those who didn't.[4] She has been particularly forceful about the use of ICU diaries to record the events that occur during an ICU stay. Providing a clear record of true memories can help erase the false memories people tend to acquire during their ICU stay. It was Jones's research that first suggested that the presence of false memories, coupled with a lack of true memories of what had happened in the ICU, contributes to post-traumatic stress disorder (PTSD) among ICU survivors.

Margaret Herridge is a dynamic and charismatic physician scientist who has established a thriving clinical and research group at the University of Toronto. Her pioneering and successful aftercare clinic has been in operation for over a decade. Herridge published many of the pivotal early papers that began to describe the outcomes people experienced after their life-threatening illnesses were treated in the ICU. She discovered that recovery often plateaued after one year, but that among people under about age 50, continued progress could be seen through at least five years after hospitalization.[5]

Dale Needham also began his work in Toronto. Now at the Johns Hopkins University in Baltimore, Needham has focused on ICU rehabilitation and—rare in American medicine—is jointly appointed in the fields of both intensive care and rehabilitation medicine. Needham runs a large and productive research group, Outcomes after Critical Illness and Surgery (OACIS), at Hopkins, now arguably the major force in the field. He has spearheaded work on early mobility and focused rehabilitation among patients in the ICU.[6]

Most researchers entered the field of ICU rehabilitation after some personal experience with a medical crisis. The details differ, but almost everyone comes through some harrowing experience that helps them identify with the plight of patients and families. Ramona Hopkins's story is particularly compelling. Thirty years ago, Hopkins was a maternity nurse and young mother. She and her husband were in their back yard, barbecuing, when a panicked neighbor interrupted the party to gesture frantically toward the driveway in front of the house. These were the years before optical sensors, and the neighbors had discovered Hopkins's four-year-old son trapped under the garage door, too small to have triggered the pressure sensor. His heart had already stopped when they extracted him from that mechanical stranglehold.

Hopkins performed CPR until the paramedics arrived, and thus began a long and dreary journey that ultimately led to their son's recovery. As she worried through his slow healing from brain injury after cardiac arrest, she found herself drawn to know more than she could as a practicing clinician. So, in the midst of helping her son to heal, Hopkins started a PhD in psychology so that she could become an expert in the brain's recovery from low oxygen. Her first attempts to start a doctoral program were met by condescension on the part of academic psychologists ("a nurse wants a PhD???"), but Hopkins rose through the academic ranks to international prominence as an expert in brain function after life-threatening illness or brain injury. It has been my personal pleasure to be mentored by her.

Together, Needham and Hopkins ran a large study to understand how survivors fare after acute respiratory distress syndrome (ARDS), one of the most common and most serious diagnoses in the ICU. Patients with ARDS may spend weeks, even months, on the ventilator and are often the sickest patients that we treat in a modern ICU. The ARDS Long-Term Outcome Study (ALTOS) has been pivotal in improving our understanding of life after life-threatening lung injury. Before ALTOS, many in the ICU community dismissed reports of PICS as speculative or irrelevant. After ALTOS, it was clear that the syndrome was real and common.[7]

These and other early researchers, especially the group at Vanderbilt University in Nashville, Tennessee, have accumulated considerable expertise, published scores of studies, and laid the groundwork for a now burgeoning field of research in outcomes after intensive care. This research has given us a much clearer vision of the challenges of life after the ICU.

POST–INTENSIVE CARE SYNDROME

We don't understand all the biological reasons for PICS yet, but we now have a decent idea of what it looks like for patients and their families.

The researchers in the field describe two forms of PICS—the syndrome affecting the person who was sick in the ICU (PICS-Patient) and a parallel syndrome that affects their family members (PICS-Family).[8] It is a little surprising at first to realize that it's not just the patient who lay in the ICU bed on life support who has new disability after an ICU stay. But increasing evidence indicates that family members are often falling apart under the stress and burdens of carrying their loved one through the crisis of a life-threatening illness.

The family syndrome of PICS is less well understood than the patient PICS. Family members are fatigued and disoriented. They remember every terrible thing that happened, every major source of stress that arose. Their thinking is often muddled, by serious anxiety, depression, or post-traumatic stress. Although the family syndrome of PICS is less well understood than the patient PICS, their suffering matters. Not only are family members deserving in their own right as individuals, but family members also become informal caregivers: The success of a patient's recovery may depend on the strength and resilience of their family members.[9]

With that caveat, it's true that patients are most affected by PICS. While researchers have developed an extensive classification for the syndrome, most of the important difficulties people encounter are related to their bodies, brains, and psyches.

Bodies

While we understand a fair bit about the body after intensive care, unfortunately what we know about those physical outcomes suggests that there's still a lot of work to do.

Many ICU survivors have limited strength and endurance. Some can't walk up a flight of stairs; others can't walk at all. Rich, who survived gallstone pancreatitis, was similar to many ICU survivors—not one of the one-third who seem to bounce back quickly and fully, but one of the two-thirds who suffer from PICS. That he is continuing to recover puts him on the more fortunate side of patients with PICS.

Some people lose limbs during their illness. When shock is severe enough, the body sometimes sacrifices arms or legs to save the heart. Gangrene can develop, leading to amputation. The need to become accustomed to a prosthetic limb or other adaptive technology adds additional difficulty to a person already weakened by the ravages of life-threatening illness. Younger patients sometimes seize the opportunity, as competitive snowboarder Amy Purdy did after she nearly died of meningitis as a teenager. While Purdy's story is unusual, her success is not unprecedented. Most people end up making do and adapting to their new disability. That's what human beings do.

The two most important of the body's problems in PICS are from damage to muscles and lungs.

MUSCLES

Almost everyone will have a measurable loss of strength in their arms and legs after intensive care, and muscle mass and strength are crucial to ultimate recovery from PICS. When people finally began surviving life-threatening illness a few decades ago, many of them were as weak as kittens. They couldn't even lift their heads off the bed, let alone stand up. This weakness dramatically slowed down their attempts to return to work and the life they lived before the illness. Critical illness neuropathy (nerve damage) and myopathy (muscle damage) contribute to the loss of strength, although simple muscle atrophy from lack of use contributes as well.

Because of the way muscles are organized, that weakness is felt particularly in the shoulders and hips—the heavy lifting muscles of the body. Many people with PICS describe their weakness more than anything as being "tired" or having low energy. They just can't keep up the same tempo they once could. For some, it feels a little like having multiple sclerosis or another chronic disease in which the muscles lack their usual power.

Researchers have tried to define what was causing this nerve and muscle damage. Was it the steroid medications doctors used as anti-inflammatories to tame the uncontrolled swelling in the lungs? Was it the strong muscle relaxers used to coordinate people's breathing with the cycles of the ventilator? Was it trouble managing the blood sugar of these sick patients? Or was it the overall medical philosophy at the time that kept people in bed in a state of suspended animation in the ICU? No one yet knows for sure.

A lot of basic research has looked at inflammation and medication effects, but so far it hasn't yielded a single clear answer. It's known that when the body is under siege, it is breaking down all its energy stores, including muscle, as part of a massive stress response. The whole body suffers during severe inflammation. Beyond that, scientists just aren't sure what causes the muscle breakdown and resulting weakness observed in so many ICU survivors.

Strict bed rest isn't helping anyone, though, which is why we encourage patients to walk around the ICU while they're still attached to the ventilator. Lying tied to a bed on a respirator with a body full of inflammatory hormones, the muscles fall apart quickly. Some evidence suggests that patients in the ICU suffer something like the muscle atrophy that astronauts experience in space. In both cases, muscles are doing unnaturally small amounts of work, whether from strict bed rest during illness or from very low gravity.[10]

The body is always tearing down and rebuilding tissue, but amid the severe physical stress of life-threatening illness, it does not engage in its normal reconstruction. Without that activity to compensate for the usual muscle losses, the muscles waste away. Interruptions in regular nutrition probably also contribute to the muscle breakdown, although a study comparing muscle strength between two different feeding strategies didn't show improvements with a more aggressive feeding schedule.[11]

The rates of loss of muscle mass are staggering. By some estimates one to two percent of muscle mass is lost every single day in the ICU. It may take a year to recover the muscle size and strength lost during a typical admission. Even though clinicians are now much more attentive to tube-feeding ICU patients than they once were (the worry was that too much food would overtax inflamed bowels; that's now considered mostly wrong), people still lose body mass as fast as people on starvation diets. Clinicians get tricked into believing that the weight loss isn't so severe because patients retain so much water as a result of weakened blood vessels.[12]

Nerves and muscles operate in a close partnership, and both are damaged during critical illness. The combination of nerve and muscle impairments may affect balance and confidence. Uneven terrain, ice or snow, and even wind may all become insuperable obstacles for ICU survivors. Some become agoraphobic and worry that they might get themselves too far from home to be able to make their way back.[13] Bicycles may be especially hard to operate, although stationary bikes and, increasingly, adult tricycles may offer some support for individuals trying to recover strength and balance. For the most severely affected, even standing may be a tall order. Ken, whose mysterious weakness after a severe infection was nearly misdiagnosed as necrotizing fasciitis, was just learning to stand again a year after his ICU admission. It would be months more before he'd be able to walk independently.

LUNGS

The same inflammation that tears down muscle tissue also erodes the fine structures of the lung, converting them to scar tissue. This process leaves many survivors' lungs extremely stiff. Seen under a microscope, the damage to the lung is astonishing. The lungs' incredibly fine network of air sacs and tiny capillaries is replaced by broken-down proteins, blood clots, and scar tissue. They look like a coastal city after a tsunami, all the support structures torn down and filled with mud and refuse. Air circulates poorly through the tangled debris, leaving many people unable to exert themselves physically. Even if the lungs can keep up with oxygen needs at rest, there's no reserve to draw on when it comes time to walk up a flight of stairs.

Along with lungs filled with biological concrete, ICU survivors commonly experience weakness of the muscles that the body uses to pump the lungs open and closed, like a bellows. Weak muscles and stiff lungs conspire to limit breathing profoundly. Rich wears oxygen because of that kind of scarring, and even if his leg muscles were strong enough, he would struggle to walk fast. If he's lucky, his body's repair systems will be able to remove enough of the scar tissue from his lungs that he'll liberate himself from an oxygen tank. But there's no guarantee, and, so far, there isn't any specific treatment beyond physical therapy. Such therapy doesn't work for everyone, and often patients can rely only on time, perseverance, and good luck.[14]

As if profound weakness weren't bad enough, patients' brains also suffer.

Brains

With the complicated exception of the liver, the brain is the only vital organ that can't be replaced with technology. With our brains we wonder and love, we pray and remember and hope. Whatever one happens to believe about the human soul, it is clearly the case that the brain is tightly coupled to consciousness. Because it is so central, the brain requires a constant supply of blood delivering sugar and oxygen. Five or six minutes without oxygen is enough to destroy the brain, while most other organs have an hour or so. During most critical illnesses, a basic level of oxygen and sugar delivery continues, but the circulation of blood drops substantially. Moreover, the chemicals and hormones the body uses to orchestrate the immune system can disrupt the blood flow within the tiniest blood vessels that feed the nerve cells deep inside the brain. The brain damage can be quite extensive: Magnetic resonance imaging (MRI) scans may show what look like multiple strokes. During the crisis, the damage within the brain manifests as delirium, that state of acute confusion so like being uncomfortably drunk.

The delirium that is so common during an ICU stay may lead to permanent, devastating cognitive impairment. More often, people suffer moderate lapses in judgment, memory, or quickness of thinking. These after-effects range from mild and transient to severe and permanent. The inability to think straight, remember new information, and efficiently make clear decisions leaves some people frankly disabled. Some highly capable people are no longer able to balance a checkbook. It's what psychologists call "executive function" that suffers the most: the ability to plan and coordinate multistep processes. Loss of memory and executive function is what is keeping Rich from returning to work. He can't keep track of all the details needed to find a pathway through his old spreadsheets and annual reports. The lucky survivors get their brains back to normal after a few months, but most ICU survivors end up with some degree of cognitive impairment for a year or more. The unluckiest may never recover.

Brian's experience started much like Rich's, although his body's failure began with swine flu. He felt feverish, and his asthma got a lot worse one day, and the next he was in the ICU on a ventilator. He spent four weeks on life support. Brian can't remember exactly when he returned to consciousness, but while he was still on substantial life support, he was awake and would shake his head and try to mouth words around the tube down his throat. (We clinicians tell people not to do it because the vocal cords flutter ineffectually and may be bruised in the process. Patients always ignore us; the hunger to communicate is too deepseated. We offer them paper on a clipboard, but they're often too weak to write clearly.)

Brian's dreams are still vivid in memory. Two main themes recurred. In one he was trapped, tied to a bed, and a faceless crowd wouldn't respond to his attempts to gain their attention. He was alone, isolated, smothering in the darkness. The other theme involved time travel. He always had a code to remember, a secret like a time capsule that would save him in the future. But he could never remember the code. In these dreams, he moved in time from the 1800s to a distant future, always anxious to remember the code that would solve the puzzle and save him. He never did, as far as he can recall. He still carries a four-week blank spot in his life that is filled with those dark dreams of isolation and broken time.

A day after he returned to consciousness, Brian was moved to a hospital ward, where elements of his nightmares became real. He lived through six endless days in which doctors and nurses seemed to appear for 60 seconds once or twice a day. He still remembers those days on the regular hospital ward as the low point in his illness. He struggled to believe that he could ever find the energy to rebuild his body's strength. He was also just beginning to process the fact that he had almost died. He was physically so weak that he didn't even notice that at the time he had the memory impairments of a person with Alzheimer's disease. Awareness of his memory difficulties increased as he recovered strength. He repeated his stories and could never quite keep track of the passage of time. He thought he was ready to return to work, but at our recommendation he undertook eight hours of cognitive assessment, followed by rehabilitation. It's been a year, and he is just now feeling like his brain has recovered the ability to think clearly. He sometimes still gets overloaded in the middle of a conversation and just has to stare into space while people go on talking around him. With time and coaching, it's slowly getting better.

It's no surprise that severe emotional trauma compounded by weak bodies and impaired brains leaves people psychologically distressed. But the extent of that distress is still striking.

Psyches

The psychological ravages associated with PICS can be as severe as the physical and mental ones. Many people leave the ICU with emotional scars as severe as those carried by combat veterans. Only a minority skate by without anxiety, depression, or PTSD or some combination of the three. While some people seem to be more resilient than others, life-threatening illness inflicts some degree of psychological stress on everyone.

Most of the research on PTSD comes from victims of war, rape, and other forms of violence. Societies used to call it "battle fatigue" or "shell shock" and just assumed that some soldiers would come back from war emotionally broken. We know substantially more about trauma and its aftermath now. With input from researchers and afflicted individuals, psychologists have developed at least a basic model of how human beings process stressful events and how acute stress can spiral into a long-term disorder.

The neural systems that can lead to PTSD are ancient; something like PTSD is probably present in some abused animals. In response to stress, structures at the base of the brain activate a complex molecular machinery. This stress response successively bathes the body in a range of chemicals and hormones. Cortisol and adrenalin are the best-known hormones, but they are just the most famous of a chemical mob.[15]

Under stress our brains become incredibly focused on any possible threats to safety. Presumably that was helpful at some point in the evolutionary past. But that response can become a serious problem in some situations, with too many frightening details to process all at once. Some researchers have called PTSD "indigestion of the brain" to highlight the reality that the traumatic experience didn't get processed, or digested, into healthy memories. The images and experiences may be so stimulating and threatening that the brain doesn't have an appropriate way to store them in the memory banks. They keep bubbling back to the surface, exacting a severe emotional price each time they do.

Part of the PTSD among ICU survivors comes from the physical illness itself, but some comes from the way ICUs are run. The immobility and the catheters, the medications to keep people calm on life support, sleep disturbances from the constant alarms and commotion at all hours of the night and day all contribute to the emotional distress and its painful echoes. A stressed-out brain can't process information normally, and benign sounds or images can be as frightening as a grizzly bear galloping toward you in the woods.

It's easy to create nightmares by accident. One former ICU patient later reported an experience in which someone—she's not sure whether it was a doctor, a nurse, a phlebotomist, a respiratory therapist, an orderly—walked quietly into her room while she was sleeping and then touched her without warning. The person was drawing blood or check-ing blood pressure or simply adjusting an oxygen monitor, and probably hoped to avoid disturbing the patient's sleep. But this young woman remembers clearly the sense of lying in her own bed and suddenly awak-ening to find an unannounced stranger staring at her and touching her arm. The ICU room had become her bedroom. She had moved in and made it her own, and the healthcare professionals were merely guests there. How would you feel, she later asked a group of clinicians trying to understand the problems of the ICU, if you were lying in your bedroom and suddenly awoke to find a stranger holding your arm? One Vietnam veteran experienced the restraints and the hospital bed as if he were tied up in the bottom of a boat. The ear thermometers his ICU nurses used felt to him like the pistol end of a game of Russian roulette played by his Viet Cong captors.

The unfamiliarity of the ICU contributes to psychological distress.[16] When there's nothing familiar to fall back on in the midst of a traumatic situation, the mind does much worse than it would otherwise. The unknown is menacing. This suggests that basic efforts to orient people to the experience of intensive care could decrease psychological dis-tress, but to date few ICUs have gone to the trouble.

Poor communication, caused by inertia, fatigue, and ignorance, clearly plays a role in psychological distress after an ICU admission. Studies from France suggest that relatively simple improvements in communication can have a substantial positive effect. A grief brochure for families and brief communication training for staff dropped PTSD rates among bereaved family members by almost half.[17] When research-ers take the time to ask, the word they hear from patients and families is that clinicians often don't meet their needs for useful information and communication.[18]

There's another side to the psychological distress that is particu-larly troubling for advance directives. Amid the sensory overload and disorientation that mark an ICU admission, participants—especially family members—must make complex decisions about the nature and extent of invasive and uncomfortable but life-sustaining treatments that are difficult to understand.[19] The burden of these decisions, par-ticularly when the framing strongly emphasizes agency and autonomy, may traumatize families, who often blame themselves for ultimate outcomes.[20] This approach to medical decisions can cast a shadow over the rest of an individual's life.[21] In my experience—corroborated by reliable studies—family members often feel that they have caused a death when they decide to stop life support; that is the burden of agency that may be unwelcome. However irrational their belief, it is nevertheless quite real for some family members who have borne alone the weight of a decision to allow a natural death to occur. Whatever the ethical issues, surrogate decision making may contribute substantially to PICS for families.

Post Intensive Care Syndrome is a labyrinth for everyone it afflicts. People encounter new challenges, new disabilities, and a medical system that is not prepared to support them in any kind of integrated way. It doesn't have to be that way. Now that we know what people face, the US medical system is starting to develop clinics, services, improved methods of communication, and new treatments. The group at Vanderbilt have been especially important in developing an ICU Recovery Center for patients and their families, a model that is beginning to extend around the United States.[22]

This rising interest in supporting survivors at times appears to be at odds with another use of research about health status after an ICU admission.

IS IT ALL WORTH IT?

What's striking in all the research on PICS is that even with the disabilities they experience, most people are still glad to be alive. They adapt. They make new lives for themselves. They thrive. The physician-researcher Brian Cuthbertson found in a study of Scottish ICU survivors that, despite typical rates of PICS, fully 80 percent were happy with their current quality of life, and every single patient was willing to undergo ICU admission again.[23]

When my research group studied patients whose shock was so severe that treatment was often deemed futile we found that about one in five of them survived. While the odds were clearly against these individuals, a 20 percent chance of survival was not what most people would call futile. Some readers of our results countered that a 20 percent chance of survival was not adequate because we didn't know what their lives looked like after surviving. This criticism implicitly assumed that the surviving 20 percent would have such low quality of life that they would be better off dead. We took that criticism to heart and tracked down the survivors to discuss with them how they were faring. We contacted them as late as five or seven years after their severe shock.

Many of these survivors had physical disabilities or were otherwise limited in some way, but the large majority of them were holding their own and thankful they survived. Their quality of life was a bit lower than their peers', but not by a dramatic margin. None of them had the dreaded "negative" health utilities, in which healthcare economists would consider them better off dead. And while our patients had some anxiety, depression, and PTSD, their overall levels of mental illness were not significantly different from those of Americans at large. The people we interviewed were all patients for whom a standard living will would have recommended death rather than perseverance: Recall that we started with a group of people so sick that care was often considered futile. These data underscore the importance of further research, activism, and rehabilitation support to help ICU survivors recover and reintegrate into society.[24]

Fatima had a rare and poorly understood crisis in the brain, peripheral nerves, and muscles that led to prolonged coma and weakness. A neurologist told her husband that, despite the uncertain cause of her unconsciousness, Fatima was in a permanent vegetative state. She had completed a standard living will that refused medical treatment in the event of permanent vegetative state, and the neurologist advocated strongly that they allow her to die.

But Fatima wasn't in a vegetative state, let alone a permanent one. The neurologist had discounted the input of nurses for the two weeks leading up to the meeting: They had witnessed Fatima occasionally attending to their presence at the bedside. The world of permanent vegetative states is full of families overinterpreting the movements of unconscious patients. In the case of Terri Schiavo, then-senator Bill Frist watched a few seconds of video and diagnosed Schiavo as not being in permanent vegetative state. She was too conscious, he argued, to let her die. Frist, a physician, was wrong; it was all political theater in retrospect, but his and similar antics have left many physicians skeptical of such reports. It's natural to discount reports that you don't see yourself, and easy to rely on your own observations and then limit those observations to just once a day. In my experience that's what some practicing neurologists tend to do. Fatima's neurologist had fallen prey to false coherence and confirmation bias. She was asleep as if in a coma, so even though there was no typical reason for her to be in the permanent vegetative state, that image dominated his thinking. I supported her family's rejection of the neurologist's advice because I thought his judgment was clouded by cognitive biases, and his interpretation of her advance directive was incorrect.

A day later, Fatima was quite visibly awake. A year after the decision to disregard the living will, she lives in a skilled nursing facility, barely able to stand. Her speech comes out a little funny. But her strength in her arms has come back fully, as have her wits. Fatima has become the life of the nursing facility, holding court with bags of candy and big smiles. The laughter floats out of her room and down the corridor. She has her tough moments, times when she is frustrated at her lack of strength and stamina and the months she lost from healthy life. She and her husband, Abdul, have discussed the decision on multiple occasions, and she is consistently glad that he didn't activate the living will. Fatima is hopeful that she will one day return home with Abdul, but she is glad to be alive even if she continues to live in a nursing home. She has benefited immensely from the increasing attention to rehabilitation after critical illness that has come with the increasing attention to PICS in recent years. I'm not taking issue with permanent vegetative state itself; once correctly diagnosed, it is exceedingly rare for consciousness to meaningfully return to individuals with permanent vegetative state. I strongly discourage life support for individuals in a permanent vegetative state. I'm suggesting that we all need to move slowly, aware of the cognitive biases that might cloud our judgment, to be sure that the diagnosis is made correctly and that patients and families are well supported regardless of the diagnosis.

The Tension between Outcomes Research and Advance Directives

While few will say it out loud, there is a generally implicit conflict between the field of ICU outcomes and the advance directives movement. While no one in the ICU outcomes world thinks people should be tortured pointlessly in an ICU or be forced to persist biologically in a state of failed consciousness, advance directives may be used in practice as a shorthand for the belief that life after the ICU is a life not worth living. That's at core why people would refuse ICU treatments: They feel that life with and after those treatments is worse than the death that will come by refusing them. By contrast, ICU outcomes researchers have come to know personally the many courageous survivors who make their way successfully through new disabilities after life-threatening illness. It's a bit perverse to use observed disability to justify death when the disabilities are measured among people who are glad to be alive.

Outcomes researchers are often mortified to discover that their careful work to describe life after the ICU is used to persuade individuals to refuse life-sustaining treatments. Anecdotally, the practice is common. Colleagues at Johns Hopkins performed an elegant study to clarify how ideas about PICS might shape decision making. The researchers asked physicians to advise hypothetical families about whether to continue life support. Researchers changed the context for the question at random: participating physicians either heard a description of the patient's values and preferences, or they were asked to imagine "functional outcomes" (a common way of talking about PICS) after the ICU. Having physicians think about PICS was far more likely to sway their opinion than thinking about the patient's values, a testimony to the moral hazards associated with current advance directives. In other words, when intensive care physicians from a national sample were primed to think about PICS, they were more likely to recommend against life support.[25] This important study sent an uncomfortable shiver down the spines of many in the field of ICU outcomes because they know individuals who have made peace with PICS and have found deep and lasting meaning in life after the ICU. The study was also disturbing because a patient's values and priorities should matter more than a physician's disability stigma when it comes to medical decisions, but they apparently did not.[26]

The conflict between the study of ICU outcomes and advance directives is tricky. When autonomy is carefully and authentically preserved, people should be able to decide that they do not want to undergo life support because it will not deliver a result acceptable to them. The idea that you can refuse medical care that won't achieve your goals or imposes a burden on you that you are unwilling to bear is fundamental to Western culture and should be supported. In life's final phases particularly, ICU treatments may only promise a deformed death.

The moral hazard for physicians and the problems with affective forecasting are relevant to the question of how to use knowledge of PICS to guide people through life-threatening illness. What worries me about the results of the Johns Hopkins study is that physicians appear to be exercising pseudo empathy by attaching their own sensibilities to the values and priorities of patients and families. It's neither accurate nor honest to suppress the fact that the large majority of ICU survivors come to flourish in their new lives. When it has been studied, the vast majority of patients with PICS—while they have disability that they would rather have avoided—don't actually wish that they were dead. As a general rule, the individual's understanding of her phase of life and values and priorities, rather than general pronouncements about PICS, should be guiding life support decisions in the ICU.

On a practical level, there is an ongoing tension between the physicians and researchers who are committed to extending the capacity of modern medicine and those who are inclined to let nature take its course. The important research in PICS must not morph into a sneak-around for clinicians to push for more rapid withdrawal of life support. There's too much risk of overriding patients' self-determination with this approach. Simultaneously, physicians ought not to paint an unrealistically rosy picture of life after the ICU. The goal of the medical system should be to support people in the well-informed pursuit of their deeply held values and priorities.

The pain and disability of PICS are real; these ICU survivors need better treatment and prevention for the ailments that beset them. There will be some individuals who would not choose to live their final months with PICS, and their decisions should be honored when clinicians have avoided bias in their communication. The work of assuring relevant communication that is tailored to authentic wishes is more difficult than reading a living will. But the moral imperative is to optimize outcomes for survivors and support everyone attentively through life-threatening illness, recognizing that our solutions have to be useful to both those who survive and those who do not.

Thanks to the patient and elegant work of a group of committed researchers willing to study something off the beaten track of molecules and genes, we now know a great deal about survival after a life-threatening illness. There is more to learn, much more, but we finally have the necessary foundation. This knowledge brings with it the responsibility to investigate ways to improve those outcomes, to make life after the ICU more livable. We can no longer assume that if people don't refuse life support we will get them through a physiological crisis and then deposit them haphazardly in an outpatient medical system and family network wholly unprepared to care for them.

Knowledge of PICS intensifies the risks of the advance directive paradigm. Inaccurate affective forecasting and the moral hazard for physicians mean there is substantial risk of clinicians using the research on PICS to stop life support for people who may have done quite well in the end and who would authentically choose that outcome if they were well supported. The field of ICU outcomes is making clear just how perilous the mistakes of the advance directives paradigm can be and pointing out areas where we can and should focus our efforts for improvement. Fortunately, such reform is slowly gaining momentum.

FUTURE

Chapter 7

Reform

The Current State of the Art

Moroni Leash, one of the pioneers of second-generation advance directives, likes to tell stories about the couples he recruited via Rotary Clubs
to practice decision making near the end of life. He interviewed wives
and husbands separately about several hypothetical scenarios in which
medical decisions would be required. In each scenario, the couples had
to decide which life support therapies they would recommend for their
spouses. Leash was testing different advance directives to see which
most improved agreement among spouses. After the couples completed
the exercise, Leash then debriefed them. These debriefing sessions
proved to be more emotional than anyone had anticipated. Not uncom-
monly he found spouses regarding each other with suspicion during the
interview. "You would force me to go through that? How dare you?" a
woman would ask her husband, eyes flashing with fury. Or, on the other
hand, a disgruntled husband complained, "What, you're trying to kill
me? You would unplug me without even trying?" People who had spent
many presumably happy decades together in marriage proved unable
to think through a few possible medical situations in which they might
make health decisions on behalf of their spouses.

Leash took those responses as proof that he was on the right path in
his efforts to develop a better, more detailed advance directive. Whether
his intuition was correct or not is a story still waiting to unfold. But
Leash's observations have been corroborated by multiple independent
studies: While we are bad at guessing what we want for ourselves, we are
even worse at predicting what loved ones believe about medical treatment when their lives are threatened.

Work by Leash and several others to improve advance directives has had varying levels of success. Some of these attempts are incremental enhancements no more useful than the original living wills, while others seek to transform the approach to helping people navigate life-threatening illness. Those that push well beyond the old paradigm of living wills hold the most promise.

ELICITING VALUES AND WISHES

In the late 1980s, the Institute for Public Law in New Mexico developed a program to provide volunteer proxy decision makers for older individuals without family members to speak for them. The New Mexico group created a Values History document meant to help those proxies better know the people they served. In addition to a few of the typical "which of these treatments do you want?" questions familiar from living wills, the Values History included several questions intended to give a sense for the texture of people's lives. What have you liked doing in life? Whom have you loved? Do you practice a specific religion or none at all?

Adding an awareness of the patient as a person is essential to providing meaningful care during life-threatening illness, and that is what the Values History has done right. Whatever becomes the ultimate solution to the problems of navigating a life-threatening illness, careful understanding and protection of the individual must be at the center of the process. Care cannot be patient-centered without knowing and honoring the person in her specificity. Still, the Values History is long and relatively unstructured—more a multi-page, do-it-yourself script for an oral history than anything else. Whether it would be better to record and transcribe an actual conversation isn't clear, but this or a similar document, plus perhaps an audio recording of conversations or stories, may be quite useful.

The Values History is not yet written in a way that would make possible mapping of the recorded values onto any particular medical decision-making strategies. Nor do the specific questions on the Values History work for everyone. But the approach—trying to understand people and where they come from rather than making them choose among hypothetical treatments they don't understand—is clearly a step in the right direction.[1]

A kindred effort came from Jim Towey, an attorney and prominent Catholic educator, who had witnessed the kindnesses shared with people dying of AIDS at Mother Teresa's Washington, DC, hospice. He felt that similar personal attention should be provided to everyone facing advanced age or terminal illness, whatever the cause. With that goal in mind, he combined a basic living will with some values elicitation and gentle instructions reminiscent of early modern *Art of Dying* texts.

Towey also seems to have recognized that the struggle over advance directives pitted proponents of euthanasia against relentless right-to-lifers in a destructive competition. Instead, he sought a middle ground, one that embraced the concept behind advance directives but maintained sensitivity to the considerations of religious and disabled people.

Towey called his new advance directive "Five Wishes," to emphasize that he wanted his living will to move beyond the simple list of options with check boxes. With it, he tried to allow for a more human-centered process rather than just culturally contentious legal documents that wrangled about the technical details of life support. The five wishes/questions of Towey's directive are:

1. Who will speak for you?
2. What treatments do you want?
3. How comfortable do you want to be?
4. How do you want to be treated?
5. What do you want your loved ones to know about you?

The first two wishes/questions are standard from other advance directives. The specific details of the third and fourth wishes have struck some observers as a bit strange, because they include a list of acts of basic comfort and kindness that almost everyone would want for themselves if they developed serious illness. What critics fail to recognize is that Towey's lists are primarily educational. They are meant as much to help inexperienced people know how to behave in the presence of the dying as to answer any specific question.

The last question nods toward values elicitation while gently suggesting the importance of life completion. The last three wishes are primarily to remind patients and their families what they ought to be doing when they face the catastrophe of a life-threatening illness. These instructions would not have been necessary before the cultural changes in the early twentieth century brought about by the Dying of Death. Despite its imperfections, the Five Wishes initiative does a decent job of providing basic instructions for navigating the end of life.

Rather than arguing categorically about the permanent vegetative state in religious terms, the Five Wishes movement proposes something of a middle ground. Through his nonprofit organization, Aging with Dignity, Towey has reached out to conservative and religious communities to advocate for moderate views about life support.[2] On the technical side, Five Wishes doesn't fix what is wrong with advance directives, but the effort improves the field by acknowledging how much else exists beyond menus of biomedical procedures. It took more creative thinking to expand advance directives further.

REGISTRATION DRIVES FOR ADVANCE DIRECTIVES IN WISCONSIN

Bernard "Bud" Hammes, a philosopher-ethicist at Gundersen Health System in La Crosse, Wisconsin, realized as early as 1991 that living wills didn't work on their own: They required an integrated system of supports for "advance care planning." The Gundersen group he led developed their own educational materials, performed community outreach, trained scores of advance care planning specialists, stationed such a specialist at every major Gundersen facility, and created a uniform documentation system. In retrospect, La Crosse provided an ideal laboratory for this kind of experiment in moving well beyond traditional advance directives. The Gundersen directives themselves were fairly similar to the documents used elsewhere, but the effort in La Crosse introduced several methodological improvements, most specifically an emphasis on hiring and training new nonphysician specialists and making advance care planning a continuous process. Their integrated advance care planning program (now commercialized as Respecting Choices®) has made waves, although it's been a struggle to make that specific system work in other environments, with the intriguing exception of Australia.[3]

The approach in La Crosse makes good sense, although the data tell a more complicated story. In the major report of the Wisconsin experience, Hammes found that while the large majority of patients had specified a proxy decision maker, only about 10 percent of people who died in the county had a living will per se.[4] Forty percent of the people who died did not require an advance directive because they were awake when they decided to allow a natural death to occur. And regardless of whether there was an advance directive, 98 percent of the deaths were "negotiated" in some way, suggesting that cultural acceptance of dying among patients and physicians in La Crosse was much more relevant than living wills. Ultimately, the major scientific finding from their report was that people tended to die in nursing homes as opposed to hospitals more often after Hammes's program had been implemented. Hammes and his colleagues did not measure the quality of dying or how well advance directives represented patients' actual desires or whether people tended to finish up their lives better, crucial oversights if the goal is better, more personalized care near the end of life.

A later follow-up report of the experience in La Crosse suggested that living wills were still rare, that Physician Orders Regarding Life-Sustaining Treatment (POLST) forms had become common and were generally complied with, and that only about 10 percent of those who requested cardiopulmonary resuscitation (CPR) actually received it. The new analysis still failed to measure more personally relevant outcomes such as quality of support received or concordance of POLST forms with patient's actual wishes.[5]

While La Crosse tends to be seen as a success story for living wills, it has actually evolved well beyond them. Their system includes not only trained educators but also an "advanced disease coordination" program, which integrates and supports the medical and personal care of people living with serious illness. These are clearly moves in the right direction. It's important not to confuse living wills with what happens in Gundersen hospitals or to imagine that a simple push to have more people complete living wills or POLST forms will achieve any-thing like what was accomplished in La Crosse. Living wills are just an echo of a much more important process, that is just now beginning to develop into something useful. Central to the Gundersen system are the substantial resources invested in personnel whose sole purpose is to improve communication between clinicians and patients and assure that patients' voices are heard in real time. Nor has the research on the Gundersen system thus far studied important, unanswered questions about the best ways to individualize guidance for people navigating seri-ous illness. Similar questions remain about how persuasive to be when presenting the options available.

MULTIMEDIA PERSUASION

One of the key problems of disclosurism is the use of legal documents to communicate. Legal documents generally only make sense to lawyers. Even as we live in a society flooded with legal documents—sometimes it feels like you can't do anything interesting without having to pretend to read a contract packed with fine print—studies clearly show that we do not read those contracts, and even if we try to read them we don't under-stand what they say.[6] If the goal is communication, legal documents are the wrong medium. But they can be efficient, and that's one of the rea-sons these documents persist. Many have felt that other mechanisms of communication are needed.

Enter video, the medium that in various formats has entertained and persuaded Americans for about a century. Since visual media are more memorable and persuasive to most people than written materials, it's reasonable to think that video could represent a middle space between live conversation and a faceless document.

Rebecca Sudore, a geriatrician in San Francisco, developed a multi-media website (www.prepareforyourcare.org) designed to help people anticipate what they and their family will need in order to make their way through serious illness.[7] In Sudore's view, it's more important to be prepared to make decisions when they arise than to make a hypotheti-cal decision long before it matters. Tasteful videos feature actors telling stories concerned with different aspects of serious illness and decision making.

Sudore's PREPARE program does an excellent job of communicating with people about what their values and choices might be and appropriately focuses on preparing people to make decisions "in the moment" or "just in time." While there's a lot more to do, PREPARE appropriately draws attention to the need to support real decisions in real time, when they happen.

Angelo Volandes, a hospitalist physician at Massachusetts General Hospital in Boston, has approached the persuasiveness of video from a different tack. Volandes developed a video series that is tied closely to the standard advance directives paradigm. Although he has worked hard to avoid bias, the clinician's moral distress often shines through in the videos.[8] Several of the videos employ a neutral-appearing, clinical format to dramatize the technical details of certain procedures and graphically portray dementia. Cardiopulmonary resuscitation is described as unlikely to work, a conclusion that inadvertently favors the views of clinicians and commentators over patients themselves. What matters most to clinicians are the mechanics of CPR and the fact that only a modest number of patients survive. What matters to most patients is their current phase of life and whether they would be forced to live as a vegetable if CPR were to fail.[9]

Video technologies work, in part, because of cognitive biases that amplify the power of a message. We pay attention to how other individuals behave and tend to model the behavior we see (psychologists call this "normativization" or "identification"). Especially when videos are produced by physicians, the moral distress physicians feel caring for individuals at high risk of death or cognitive disability bleeds over into the communication. Thus, Volandes's group has performed multiple studies demonstrating that if they show people a video that presents CPR, without relevant life context, as a procedure that rarely works, then people are less likely to choose it.[10] A less stark video developed at the Mayo Clinic did not on average change people's code status decisions. The Mayo Clinic's video clearly improved patients' knowledge of the mechanics of CPR but did not induce people to change their minds. This comparison offers an important reminder of the influence of even unintentional bias and the risks that the traditional advance directive paradigm can undercut autonomy.[11]

Videos can make end-of-life issues vivid, but they don't make the living will any more useful or applicable if our goal is to honor the values and priorities of individual patients. The videos are still tied to the deeply flawed infrastructure of advance directives. Without solving the underlying problems, making living wills more persuasive through video is not the right solution. Given the disturbing evidence that many people who have Do Not Resuscitate (DNR) or Do Not Intubate (DNI) orders don't actually want to be DNR or DNI, I worry that persuasive videos will only make more people sign orders that they do not understand for medical decision they don't actually endorse.

For multimedia-supplemented advance care planning to actually enhance autonomy, the multimedia tools must inspire and enable conversations between physicians (or well-trained facilitators) and patients while avoiding the inadvertent biases of living wills. As long as videos are tied to the old system, it is unlikely that they will lead to more and better conversations, because physicians feel busy and the old system amplifies their biases. A new system may employ videos and other multimedia methods, but the goal will be to improve communication and the tailoring of information to the individual person. Substantial work remains to be done.

TAILORING ADVANCE CARE PLANNING

Advance directives aspired to respect individual wishes, but stock general forms don't fulfill that aspiration. What's needed instead is specific relevance to the actual details of a person's life. Bud Hammes's group in Wisconsin rightly advocates tailoring advance care planning to such situations, perhaps the most important of his methodological developments. People need personalized, highly relevant guidance during life-threatening illness. So far they've had limited access to such options.

However they were initially intended, advance directives are not primarily designed to make our experience of life-threatening illness more healthful. If they do so, it is a happy accident. In my experience, people want honest, accurate communication about a specialist's best estimates of what phase of life they are living and then support for the meanings that can be created during that phase. For the rare individuals who have strong, highly specific opinions about medical procedures, advance directives may allow some of their preferences to be honored. Most people care mainly about the quality of their lives, receiving honest communication, and whether a proposed plan of care might or might not fulfill their goals.

The image of a guide is again important here. Guidance does not mean dictating outcomes or paternalistically forcing a specific point of view, but walking with people along a difficult and unfamiliar path. Clinicians should strive to be such guides, able to customize a plan to the individual's needs. Effective guides are open to what the individual values and prioritizes, aware of how the individual thinks, and able to help the individual understand whether there are threats to autonomy or personhood that may need to be confronted. Intensive, rigorous research in large groups of patients is required to create the maps that will show the path from an individual's sensibilities, values, and priorities to specific medical plans. So far, there's a giant void in medical understanding of authentic personalization, and this lack of understanding creates a serious barrier to robust expressions of autonomy.

Because it's not just priorities that differ but also medical situations—advance care planning must be specific to a person's anticipated future. If you have advanced emphysema, for example, you'll need guidance relevant to what tends to happen in late emphysema. While some diseases overlap near the end, patients with advanced heart failure will have different events to anticipate and decisions to ponder than patients with breast cancer. The first step is to know, for each individual, what is likely to come next. Once that's reasonably settled, the next step is to identify and understand personal preferences relevant to that expected future. When approaches to decisions are made explicit and systematic, they are called decision aids.

Decision Aids

Over the last thirty years, a field of medical research has emerged, focused on the mechanics of decisions. These researchers have distilled their findings into "decision aids," which are meant to guide people through the process of making a medical decision. Decision aids are formal protocols, often on paper but increasingly in electronic formats, that collect input from users and guide them through their options, including the associated trade-offs. As opposed to video-enhanced advance directives, which make old-school advance directives more powerful, decision aids begin the work of guiding individuals through decisions in ways that incorporate patients' values and priorities. The evidence suggests that when people use decision aids, they tend to feel they have made better decisions.[12]

Some of the earliest and most successful decision aids were related to prostate cancer screening and treatment. Should I watch and wait, patients wondered, or is surgery the answer? If surgery, how extensive, and should it involve radiation? What side effects should I worry about? Other early decision aids tried to help women decide how to proceed when they were diagnosed with early stage breast cancer, in which several medically equivalent options have different side effects.[13]

Researchers at Dartmouth Medical School and the University of Ottawa have done perhaps the most extensive work in developing and testing decision aids. Among the aids developed at Ottawa, one helps parents choose whether to get a second cochlear implant for their child and one guides patients deciding whether to undergo ultrasound treatment for knee arthritis. Some of the decision aids are educational tools intended to persuade people not to engage in unproven or risky treatments, while others are meant to bring patients into full partnership with their clinicians. Ottawa has even developed a specific decision aid for patients in the ICU and another one for people with advanced lung disease. In addition to the aids they have developed themselves, Ottawa keeps a list of perhaps a hundred, including ten on prostate cancer alone, that have been developed by researchers around the world.[14]

Decision aids work best when mortality doesn't figure too prominently in the deliberations. However helpful these aids are in navigating the course of various diseases, human feelings about death and suffering often don't fit well into the quantitative terms on which most decisions aids are based. Filling out a computerized question-naire while coping with a serious illness, even a form that is well con-ceived, may not help us scrutinize what kinds of risks balance against what kinds of benefits when it comes to the timing of our death. With those limitations in mind, Christopher Cox has been leading an effort at Duke University to develop and test a decision aid for people con-fronting more than a week on the ventilator, people who will soon meet the criteria for chronic critical illness. In early studies, Cox's decision aid helped physicians and family members understand each other and come to agreement more quickly, without evidence of clinician bias shaping the decisions.[15]

Ultimately, if decision aids are going to improve outcomes for people with serious illness, they will need to offer valid, personalized advice and map a person's insights onto relevant medical decisions. Two professors of medicine and humanities at Penn State, Benjamin Levi and Mike Green, have developed an interactive electronic deci-sion aid they call Making Your Wishes Known. While working on a PhD in philosophy, Levi developed a dialogue-based model of autonomy that focused on conversations as a way to support self-determination.[16] Working with Green, Levi then developed a sys-tem with sophisticated logic to guide people through the process of advance care planning. They've been able to show in early tests that people with advanced cancer aren't upset by using the computer pro-gram, and people's responses to the "big picture" questions within the system don't change from month to month.[17]

I suspect that the best possible chance for an approach like tradi-tional advance care planning will be through something like what Levi and Green are doing. They ask interrelated questions to build a draft advance directive and then ask the user to decide whether the proposed directive makes sense. There's still more work to do, and their system is still trying to tie individuals to prespecified hypotheticals. But the Making Your Wishes Known program is making strides toward more serious individualization of advance care planning. Any such system will need to deal with our predictable irrationalities, but this doesn't mean we can't use careful thinking to improve the process of honoring individuals in their specificity.[18]

Choice Architecture

Thanks to behavioral economics, which has challenged the idea that people are perfectly rational or should be expected to be, cognitive psychology has become standard fare in the media and in water cooler conversation. Especially following the work of scholars like Richard Thaler and Cass Sunstein, the authors of the popular book *Nudge*, people are acknowledging that there isn't solid evidence behind the old idea that people make decisions the way economics textbooks used to think they did.

Behavioral economists have seized on "choice architecture" as a key tool for changing behavior, a technique marketers have been using for centuries. It describes the different ways in which choices can be presented to individuals—usually consumers—and the impact of a particular type of presentation on decision making. As one example among many, decreasing the size of plates or drinking cups in a cafeteria will encourage people to eat and drink less.

Some researchers are advocating choice architecture to improve advance care planning. Scott Halpern, a physician-researcher at the University of Pennsylvania, founded the Fostering Improvement in End-of-Life Decision Science center in large part to apply choice architecture to decisions about the end of life. Halpern's group performed an intriguing study. They randomly distributed one of three different versions of the standard Pennsylvania living will to individuals who had a short life expectancy. The only difference among the three living wills was which preference came first on the document. They found that about one in five participants might have made a different selection merely as a result of the default order of options on the form they received.

Halpern's group concluded that many people do not hold strong preferences about end-of-life treatments. They did not discuss the likelier possibility that living wills are inadequate instruments for measuring such preferences. People do have strong preferences about how they wish to be treated when their lives are threatened; they just don't know how to map those preferences onto current living wills. That study didn't suggest that changing defaults will improve living wills, it suggested that living wills don't communicate well.

Even with choice architecture, the risk that clinician and policy maker bias will strong-arm patients remains high. The more sophisticated approach of choice architecture bears much of the same risk as the current system. The moral hazard that affects physicians can sway choice architects just as easily. In fact, the risk of that moral hazard increases substantially, because entire populations may be affected by the choices of such architects. As with video presentations, choice architecture makes a point of view more persuasive. However, if the point of view is misleading or poorly fitted to the problem at hand, the greater persuasion can be quite risky.

The basic idea behind choice architecture is to make it easier for people to do the right thing: quit smoking, eat vegetables, recycle soda cans. But none of us knows what the right thing is during a given life-threatening illness. The whole point of self-determination is that everyone is different. One size does not fit all. Clinicians, researchers, and policy makers have strong opinions, but they often poorly reflect the values and priorities of individual patients. In the case of serious illness, the task of choice architecture should be to help people make decisions in ways that are most authentic to them as people, not in ways that are most consistent with the opinions of policy makers.

Important modifications of this approach may be able to move us to the next level, using choice architecture to help people achieve the ends *they* desire. Choice architecture at the end of life should be tailored to the individual's notion of the good life. There is still substantial mapping left to do, and far more research in order to understand what people actually want, but there is still a glimmer of hope in the insights of behavioral economics.

THE SCIENCE OF COMMUNICATION

The physician-ethicist Doug White has spent a career seeking to understand how family members make decisions on behalf of their distressed loved ones. He has used simulations and video recordings of family meetings—those special sit-down encounters where physicians provide updates and/or guidance about the next steps to take during a life-threatening illness—as a window on these complicated acts of communication. He has clarified, in great detail, what actually occurs during family meetings and how participants understand them.

White's group has done extensive, careful work to understand what is happening in the minds of people participating in decision making during an ICU admission. They have launched a "Four Supports" study to see whether providing special access to a nurse trained in communication will improve the process of decision making. Four Supports is enrolling participants in the study now and should have results to report by 2020. This program is what the Study to Understand Prognoses and Preferences for Outcomes and Risks of Treatment (SUPPORT) of the early 1990s should have been—theoretically sophisticated and focused on the experience of decision making rather than clinician-oriented outcomes like code status designations.

Randy Curtis's group at the University of Washington in Seattle has also done important work on communication in the ICU. Coming mostly from the perspective of palliative care and a focus on the end of life, Curtis's group has developed ways to measure the quality of death and dying and tested several interventions to improve the quality of communication in the ICU. His team performed a study that approached communication as a question of relationships, using the psychological theory of attachment. This theory maintains that people have specific styles of connecting with other people, styles that begin early in childhood and stay consistent through adulthood. Often, if you can identify a person's attachment style, you can adopt a communication strategy that is appropriate to that style. Curtis's group, like White's, used trained professionals to enable communication. Their study suggested that participants had less depression and with no higher mortality, patients died after about a week as opposed to after four weeks.[19]

Curtis's research is responsible for the important if commonsensical observation that families in the ICU rated as most satisfactory the meetings in which they spent more of the time talking.[20] People tend to listen with their mouths, and Curtis correctly pointed out the need to hear family during those meetings rather than just explain. After Curtis published these observations, I changed my practice and now try to start meetings with questions, provide extra opportunities for families to have input, and allow them to do more talking. It wasn't natural at first—I find myself wanting to fill in silences or speak quickly. But with time, I've been learning to be quieter.

Critical care physicians may be able to learn from cancer clinicians. The oncology clinic and the ICU are quite similar. In both settings, unwanted farewells are distressingly common. Simultaneously, doctors and patients harbor real and sometimes valid hopes for better and longer life, even when they come with the cost of often painful treatments.[21] Susan Block, a palliative care psychiatrist at Harvard, has led several efforts to improve serious illness communication among patients with cancer. Her group of collaborators at the Dana Farber Cancer Institute have observed that patients who had discussions about the end of life while undergoing treatment for cancer did better than those who did not.[22] These observations and others have led to the identification and testing of rigorous methods to be sure that such conversations happen when they should.[23] Recognizing that living wills are entirely inadequate to the tasks at hand, Block, in collaboration with Atul Gawande at Ariadne Labs, is currently wrapping up a large study of cancer patients for their Serious Illness Care program in which participants are randomized to special communication supports that are designed to serve them in their specificity as they walk through the valley of shadows. Parallel efforts are exploring the best methods to support individuals confronting life on dialysis or chronic critical illness.

I've seen firsthand the power of timely discussions and the difficulties the current system has in accommodating such discussions. For many people, it's the luck of having a physician friend that gets them through.

Jeff Valentine[24] was a tax accountant who loved muscle cars and looked out for me after my dad was gone. A kind of surrogate father, he had an outsize influence on my adolescence in semirural Utah in the 1980s. Around age fifty, Jeff developed multiple myeloma, a cancer of bone marrow that eats away at bones and weakens the immune system. Chemotherapy and a couple of bone marrow transplants followed. I saw Jeff and his wife Doris periodically over the years as he slowly weakened. He became unsteady on his feet and a little slower under the influence of the narcotic pain medications that held the groaning of his weakening skeleton down to a steady buzz rather than clanging cymbals. My family and I moved back to Utah toward the end of his journey with myeloma. Jeff and Doris would stop by my clinic to say hello when they came to the hospital for their oncology appointments.

Doris called one day to say that they'd had enough of aggressive medical treatment. Jeff had been admitted to the hospital with sepsis and dehydration, neither requiring life support. The myeloma was back in full swing, and the oncologists felt it was time for another bone marrow transplant. Jeff and Doris needed an honest answer from a knowledgeable friend about whether they had reached a clinical crossroads. No advance directive applied in their circumstance, but they were struggling.

I reviewed the situation and spoke with Jeff and Doris at length. After our conversation, we agreed that they were in fact at a crossroads. Jeff went on hospice a few hours later. I'm convinced that the myeloma oncologist would have respected an advance directive when Jeff reached the point of formal life support. But by choosing a transition to hospice when they did, Jeff got to be home for a few hours and was able to say goodbye to his family. After those first few hours he became restless, short of breath, and confused.

While hospice often works well, in this case an overburdened hospice nurse hadn't thought through next steps carefully with Jeff's family. Doris asked me to come by and help as Jeff became uncomfortable. They had thousands of dollars of medical equipment but hadn't been taught how to give Jeff's medicines for anxiety and pain under his tongue. I showed her how to use the eyedropper to administer the medications, and Jeff settled down quickly. He died peacefully before dawn.

In Jeff's case, he and Doris had been able to communicate about important issues before the loss of consciousness, independent of any formal advance care planning. Such conversations outside medical settings are critical, and they are finally receiving the attention they deserve.

THE CONVERSATION PROJECT

When the celebrated journalist Ellen Goodman retired, she turned her energies to the Conversation Project, which brings together a diverse team of experts and opinion leaders to create systems to help people talk about their priorities regarding medical care when death may be near. Goodman was driven by experiences during her own mother's slow decline to draw attention to the centrality of personal relationships and conversations rather than just legal forms at this vulnerable phase of life. The Conversation Project focuses on a key element that has been missing from reform efforts—social change must support legal and medical solutions and vice versa.

I love Goodman's emphasis on conversation rather than legalistic menus of hypothetical medical procedures. Even if we do not choose which treatments we might accept or refuse when death may be near, having conversations about our mortality can be healthy, even beautiful.

Goodman and her board recognized that it takes two to tango— people need to be having conversations, and healthcare facilities need to be ready to honor the conversations that have occurred. The Conversation Project has tasked hospitals and healthcare systems with being "conversation ready." To date, this has meant developing methods to archive and retrieve typical advance directives. Hospitals that are working to become conversation ready have started to do a portion of what Bud Hammes and his colleagues implemented in Wisconsin, developing programs to make patients' priorities visible to clinicians at every visit.

Goodman has managed to recruit some very smart people to her team, and they battle constantly against the perception that advance directives are the main point, recognizing that, ideally, advance directives are just traces of much more important conversations. It's a tough problem because so many moving parts—computer systems, culture, ethics, and medical organization—all play a role. If not done carefully, becoming "conversation ready" may just intensify problems in current approaches. Whether such a system can work without the facilitators that Bud Hammes has used is an open question. Additional study will be required, but the Conversation Project and its push to make hospitals conversation ready looks to be a substantial improvement. Just as important, we will need maps from the conversations people have to specific treatment plans in actual medical systems. Those maps do not yet exist, but Goodman's Conversation Project, in combination with the rigorous techniques being evaluated in Ariadne Labs' Serious Illness Care Program, represent excellent progress.

It's important, even with approaches like the Conversation Project, to avoid a false dichotomy. A sharp focus on the end of life is a problem in the ICU. The problem of humanizing the ICU isn't all about death. It can't be. The false belief that a given patient is either fighting for life or dying has caused too many blind spots and missteps. Solutions need to be workable for both those who ultimately survive and those who die, because we generally don't know what ultimately awaits at the time treatments are being delivered.

REDESIGNING THE INTENSIVE CARE UNIT

The Gordon and Betty Moore Foundation has taken another tack. The Intel founder's philanthropic foundation started funding research in environmental conservation and basic science in 2000. At the urging of Betty Irene Moore, the foundation began supporting improvements in patient care a few years later, with a focus on Northern California, including the founding of the Betty Irene Moore School of Nursing at the University of California, Davis.

Building on its successes in California, in 2012 the Moore Foundation established a formal program to improve the experience and outcomes of healthcare, with an initial focus on eliminating preventable harms. Recognizing the intense threats to personhood associated with an ICU admission and attracted by important research at top medical centers, the Moore Foundation became interested in reengineering how intensive care is delivered by using a systems approach. They enlisted researchers at Johns Hopkins University, Beth Israel Deaconess Medical Center, Brigham and Women's Hospital, and the University of California, San Francisco, in a collaborative effort to redesign the ICU.

The foundation proposed that the techniques and technologies of engineering, integrated with the work of physician researchers from academic medicine, could change the very structure of the ICU. This ambitious project brought together PhDs, MDs, social workers, anthropologists, nurses, physical therapists, engineers, business analysts, and computer scientists to eliminate preventable harm in the ICU.

The foundation also recognized that harms to people in hospitals are not just medical and expanded the definition of preventable harm to include the loss of respect and dignity experienced by patients and their families. In parallel with its work in the ICU, the foundation developed the "Roadmap for Patient + Family Engagement in Healthcare" to explore ways that healthcare professionals could partner with people in their medical care.[25]

I'm fortunate, as a collaborator with the team at Beth Israel Deaconess Medical Center, to work with this distinguished group of clinicians and researchers. Already, participating sites have patients more awake and mobile on the ventilator, communicating more openly about their values and priorities, and families are participating more directly in bedside care. Sites are breaking down barriers to participation of patients and families at every level of the healthcare system. These early efforts point toward a bright future.

BUILDING PARTNERSHIPS TO SUPPORT FLOURISHING

We're also witnessing a crucial transformation in the way life after the ICU is perceived. While the movement began in Europe and Canada, the United States is finally starting to focus on providing useful aftercare for patients and families recovering from an ICU admission. Typical problems with the organization of American healthcare have limited the reach of such activities in the past, but large groups of clinician-researchers are breaking new ground. I've already mentioned the Vanderbilt Recovery Center, which is leading the pack in the United States. They coordinate medical care, make sure that hospital discharge plans are carried through, provide support and counseling, and work to nurture their patients along the road to recovery. Other groups are following their lead. While a huge amount of research needs to be done to understand what changes will be most useful to people after ICU admission, the enthusiasm is building.

In 2014 the Society of Critical Care Medicine, the main organization for intensive care professionals in the United States, formed the "Thrive" Task Force to develop new methods for involving survivors directly in the critical care community. This Task Force is working hard to improve life for people after the technological drama of the ICU has ended and the slow path toward recovery has begun. Thrive's early work has focused on building communities and support networks for survivors, ways for them to band together as they navigate a medical system that is only now learning how to be useful to them. Several other organizations have undertaken similar projects, evidence of growing interest in using the scientific understanding of PICS to improve medical and personal care for people who have survived an ICU admission. Sustained, sincere partnerships are crucial to guiding patients and families through the maze of life after an ICU admission.

As important as partnership is in the life of individual patients and their families, it's not enough to partner only at the level of the individual patient. Experienced patients and families ought to be contributing to the design of healthcare organizations and systems as well. While various models are still being tested, Patient-Family Advisory Councils (PFACs) have begun to show how such partnerships might function. The work of PFACs began in pediatric hospitals, where parents have a dominant role in the interactions between patients and clinicians; within PFACs, parents collaborated with administrators and medical leaders to shape hospital policies. For pediatricians, PFACs have become par for the course. Beth Israel Deaconess Medical Center has been a pioneer in the effort to bring PFACs to adult hospitals, particularly ICU environments. Through their PFACs, they have made material differences in how their ICUs operate. Following their lead, our group started an ICU-specific PFAC at Intermountain in 2013. Knowing that we are accountable to actual patients and families for the progress we make in humanizing the ICU has encouraged us to think and act more clearly and responsibly. Our PFAC advisors tell us what is broken in our current approaches and offer possible solutions that wouldn't occur to health professionals. Perhaps most importantly of all, these advisors break down the walls that normally separate clinicians from the people they serve.

If we're smart about it, the next decade may deliver an efflorescence of healthful change. Many current efforts hold promise, although important gaps remain. Regardless, it is time to rethink at a fundamental level how ICUs are structured and operated. The community needs to learn to guide patients and families through the valley of shadows associated with a life-threatening illness.

As we reform the medical system, we need to be attentive to what is likely to work and what is less likely to represent true improvement. The state of the art includes a variety of options and ideas. Some of them are the early phases of great ideas—the Conversation Project, the Moore Foundation work, and the Making Your Wishes Known initiative. Others are mostly intensifications of the basic advance directives, especially videos that aren't integrated into an overall effort to honor autonomy robustly.

We need better methods for identifying clinical crossroads and defining what is actually at stake in a given medical decision. We need to move beyond legalistic fights about which specific procedures might be performed at which moment in time. We have to extend the conversations outside medicine and into general society. We need to figure out ways to live powerfully and authentically in the face of death. We need more people involved to recognize the communities large and small that can and should be involved in our lives during life-threatening illness. We need maps that will help people navigate the journey from values and priorities to technical medical decisions.

We need to heal the ICU.

Chapter 8

Healing the Intensive Care Unit

I received an unexpected e-mail a couple of years ago from Spence, a young man whose wife I had recently treated. He told me,

> Beyond using your medical skills to treat her physical problems, you went out of your way to make sure my questions and concerns were taken care of. You spent extra time talking with me and giving me honest assessments and advice. When she returned to consciousness you again took the time to talk with us about her experience, helped us understand what to expect and what recovery would be like. In other words, you treated us, and especially her, like an individual. She wasn't another body in a bed and I wasn't another shadow in the corner.[1]

Call me maudlin, but I felt the rush of warmth in my face that heralds tears when I read that paragraph. I took care of Kristi after I had already spent a year developing the Center for Humanizing Critical Care, and she and her husband Spence were one of the first couples to experience our integrated efforts at personalized, humane care in the ICU. They were a special case, not just because they came shortly after the Center's work was underway but also because they were parents of young children.

I've been practicing medicine long enough now that I have become reasonably expert at providing critical care to a wide range of patients, and the procedures no longer frighten me the way they sometimes did when I was in training. But pregnant women and young parents still scare me a little as a clinician. When I treat parents of young children, I feel the weight not just of those patients' fates but of their children's lives as well.

A few days after the birth of her third child, Kristi developed a pneumonia gone wild. The inflammation of an immune system out of control caused her lungs to fill with fluid, her blood pressure to plummet, and her kidneys to fail. She had a classic case of multiple organ dysfunction syndrome (MODS), a condition I have treated and studied for years. Hers came as a result of a serious Strep infection. I have learned to respect that disease and have seen many patients die from it despite all our best medical treatments. Nationally, almost half of patients with the MODS will die.

When we had to transition Kristi to life support on her first day in the ICU, I told Spence to hope for a positive outcome but acknowledged there was a chance that Kristi would not survive. Before I intubated Kristi, I encouraged Spence to tell her how much he loved her and how much he was cheering for her recovery. I knew that after intubation she would lose the ability to communicate, at least temporarily, and did not want to steal what could be last words of love from them.

In many patients with lung injury after a recent pregnancy, it is difficult to maintain oxygen levels, and Kristi's levels could barely stay adequate during her intubation, making the procedure far more stressful than usual. Still, the tube went in, and the ventilator took over her breathing. I provided Kristi's family with updates each day and made sure that when I reviewed labs or made clinical assessments I did so in her room with her family. At least once a day, I spoke with the family about how they were coping and specifically urged them to take time to go for walks, eat decent food, and get a good night's sleep now and again. And I tried to keep misinformation to an absolute minimum as our team communicated with them.

There was never any question in my mind about how hard we would fight to save Kristi's life. I knew that we would move mountains to do so. But I also knew that she might not survive despite our best efforts, and in either case, she and her family were at high risk for psychological distress. I knew that both the severity of her illness and the ways we behaved could contribute to psychological harm. It was the second harm, from poor support, that I see now as inexcusable. That was what my team and I worked to prevent. We tried to treat Kristi and Spence the way I wish my wife, Kate, and I had been treated when we were the patient and family.

It took Kristi two weeks to recover to the point that she could communicate and remember conversations. Once she was breathing on her own and clearheaded, we all began to relax. As our hope for recovery became more secure, our conversations became lighter, more focused on convalescence and rehabilitation. At that point, Spence took me aside and asked me whether I had sugarcoated my communications with him. He'd overheard nurses doing signout one evening, and one updated the other by saying, "She looks like shit." That blunt phrase had set Spence to wondering whether I had been giving him false hope during our conversations.

At her worst, Kristi had about a one-in-three chance of dying as a result of her illness, and I was honest about those estimates with Spence during our daily updates. The nurses were also giving their honest assessments, but their moral distress had made them unduly pessimistic.

Kristi's outcome was the best we could have hoped for: full recovery of body and mind, and no obvious psychological harm inflicted by the systems of care. Unfortunately, while medical successes like Kristi's are increasingly common, most people carry deep scars from an ICU experience. Many of those scars could have been prevented. No one will ever be able to remove entirely the pain of life-threatening illness, but medical professionals are morally responsible for eliminating the needless suffering of patients and their families.

Through our work on reform I have come to realize that I contributed to these problems in the past, and I am ashamed. When I'm tired or overloaded or distracted I still fall short. It would be easy to see this as a problem of some recalcitrant physicians with poor bedside manners. That's an easy but useless way out of our current bind. It's not a question of relying on ICU clinicians to have a specific passion for making sure people are not "bodies in a bed" or "shadows in a corner." While that would be ideal, it's unrealistic to expect that every physician will be great with people. Nor is disclosurism the answer to the present moral crisis.

Efforts to improve the ICU experience and replace advance directives should provide a cultural context in which life-threatening illness and death can be meaningfully interpreted, honor and acknowledge people in their diversity, create useful maps between people's individual values and priorities and specific patterns of decision making, and employ multiple, complementary approaches to improving conditions in both medicine and society.

Ultimately, new approaches will solve the problems that living wills were meant to address, at which point living wills in their current form will go away. The repaired ICU will incorporate systems to help patients and physicians understand how they can move from an individual's sensibilities and aspirations to specific technical medical decisions. A humanized ICU will train clinicians and probably others to serve as personal guides for patients and families through serious illness.

In this chapter I think through three parallel considerations: changes in medicine, social changes, and how best to replace advance directives. What unites these strategies is the attempt to frame solutions in terms of the patient's perspective rather than allowing the needs of clinicians and policy makers to dominate. What I'm advocating is the development of systems that allow human beings to flourish even in the face of serious illness in ways that are attentive to what people actually want and aspire to. I describe several ideas here; many more are possible.

LET FAMILIES IN

Humanizing the ICU requires that medical professionals acknowledge that they can heal or harm people beyond their individual patient. Historically, the medical system has focused exclusively on the individual patient lying in the ICU bed. But when life is threatened, people rely heavily on and are represented by networks of people who love them. The exclusive spotlight on the patient has caused collateral damage, and a humane ICU will support an expanded vision of "patient," one that includes families.[2]

This does not mean risking harm to the patient or keeping the patient in the dark to satisfy inappropriate requests from a family member. Rather, it means understanding families and guiding them through the experience of an ICU admission. I don't mean to gloss over the fact that some families are dysfunctional or that some individuals lack families entirely. In those circumstances, clinicians and the medical system will have extra responsibilities. The key point is that clinicians should not disrupt people's networks of trust and strength.

Relatively immediate changes include establishing Patient-Family Advisory Councils (PFACs), opening up visiting hours, and making ICU diaries available for patients and families. In my view, a PFAC should be a standard component of any substantial ICU. The voices of actual patients and families should be heard.

Outdated ideas about whether people should be stimulated while they're sick in the hospital, combined with the old culture of medical parentalism, have left too many ICUs still hostile to visitors. When my close friend's father lay dying in an ICU in South Carolina in 2014, his large family heard from staff that no more than two of them were allowed to be at his side for no more than 20 minutes at a time, up to five times per day. While that hospital's policy was particularly backward, the fact that such rules could still be on the books at this late date is frankly irresponsible.[3] This same logic kept partners out of delivery rooms during childbirth for decades, what was in retrospect an intolerable practice. Partners have appropriately become an expected fixture during childbirth, even in operating rooms where babies are delivered via cesarean section surgery. People sick enough to be admitted to the ICU want, need, and deserve the presence of their families at least as much as people giving birth. That some ICUs still routinely restrict visitation should be deeply embarrassing to the entire medical system.

Fortunately, an increasing number of ICUs has embraced open visitation; the time is long overdue to open every ICU for family visitation. Whenever the issue has been studied, open visiting hours have been either neutral or positive; one Italian study suggested fewer heart problems among patients who were allowed to receive visitors without restriction. Intensive care units should be open to visitors as dictated by the patient's desires and occasional procedures. Anything less constitutes a moral failure. With very rare exceptions for the safety of the patient, I personally allow families to stay, even during the procedures I perform, as long as they and the patient want them there (about half do in my experience).[4] Having families by my side has changed my experience dramatically, for the better. I find that our communication is better, their stress is lower, and our sense of working together as a team is heightened. Hard conversations about death come naturally when we have always been working as a team.

The ICU diary, a day-by-day account of events, written in collaboration by clinicians and family members, is the most successful intervention to decrease psychological distress among ICU survivors. Because false memories are common, patients need help reassembling what happened to them while they were unconscious. Such ICU diaries allow families to document the true memories so that they can share them with the patient later. These diaries can be deeply collaborative affairs, with everyone contributing snippets of news, or more personal, with just a spouse completing daily entries. Within our work for the Moore Foundation, we're building electronic ICU diaries, but even a cheap notepad will do. The evidence is now sufficient in my view that people shouldn't be admitted to the ICU anymore without being at least offered the option to keep an ICU diary.[5]

I'm convinced that even these three simple steps—creating PFACs, open visitation, and ICU diaries—will do more to humanize the ICU than any living will could. These steps emphasize sustained collaboration and interventions that address psychological needs beyond just acute decision making. These are just the three that do not need more research and development. They are only the beginning, though: Many more steps remain to be taken.

FIXING CODE STATUS

It would be too easy to feel tense about the failures of the current system or the urgency of reform and thus to rush headlong into solutions that don't work well. That sort of zeal without knowledge is how we ended up with advance directives in their current forms, including "code status" designations.

The risk of rushing applies at both the societal and personal levels, on scales both large and small. In my experience, physicians in training feel an urgency to settle the question of code status right at the time of admission. That urgency is usually misplaced. I've watched trainees become absolutely frantic when they hand off the care of a patient to another trainee for the night, trying to decide what the precise code status will be. The urgency they feel leads them to broach important questions in a mad rush, with no context or preparation. After asking a few questions to hone the diagnosis and doing a cursory physical examination, the young physicians commonly ask of the patient, "Now, if your heart stops, should we try to restart it?"

These rushed discussions about "code status" at the moment of admission are like meeting someone in a bar and immediately asking, "Will you be my life partner?" It's just too abrupt. I've heard enough complaints from patients and families over the years to know how a large number of people experience the process. "Good heavens," many think, "What aren't you telling me about my heart?" Or "Why aren't they committed to helping my father recover?"

These disturbing conversations with physician trainees are a direct outcome of the Patient Self-Determination Act (PSDA) of 1990 and its requirement that hospitals document advance directives at the time of admission. In retrospect this requirement forced hospitals to comply with a poorly conceived solution to an important problem and they rushed to the most resource-efficient method. The grand aspirations of the PSDA have boiled down to cursory and confusing discussions about "code status" held with untrained residents an hour after hospital admission.[6] While it's best to have phases-of-life conversations as an outpatient with a trusted clinician, there will always be more to clarify in the hospital. So it's worth getting the hospital conversations right.

Our team has spent the last three years working on this problem and discovered several things. Tricky discussions about the possibility of death need to come in context and need to be framed in terms that make sense to people. I rarely ask directly about "code status" or CPR anymore, waiting until our conversations or the patient's physiology make such procedural questions necessary. In my experience, most people are somewhere close to "full code" until they feel they are in life's final phase and want an exclusive focus on comfort rather than life prolongation once their medical condition deteriorates beyond reasonable prospects of recovery. Most people, until they are at peace with the fact that their life is near its end, want a trial of treatments. That's generally "full code" in the current system. Most people who say they aren't full code are actually just trying to refuse life in a vegetative state, not CPR itself.

To give the relationship some time to mature, I now follow a "third visit" rule for conversations about the patient's phase of life. I don't guide conversations toward questions about whether to refuse some medical procedures until I've had two previous meetings with patients and their families. Those first visits are devoted to the medical problems at hand and to getting to know each other better. I watch closely during those initial visits to see how patients and their family members react to good news and bad. I listen for clues that they feel that life is naturally near its end. I learn about their health before the crisis. I ask them how they like to communicate. And I demonstrate that I am fully committed to providing the best possible medical care, both technological and humane. It's been my experience that by our third such encounter most people are willing and able to have an honest, illuminating conversation about whether to entertain limits to heroic medical treatments.

When a patient is perilously ill, we may have three visits in two hours. When a patient is less sick, it may take two days before we have the conversation. Because of the close relationship between severity of illness and frequency of visits, I have found my "third visit" rule to work well in a wide variety of clinical situations, even if at times I push the discussion a little earlier or a little later, depending on the individual.

It's okay to take your time. Unanticipated cardiac arrests are generally the most treatable. Sudden problems with the heart's rhythm, a popped lung, or sudden severe bleeding are the kinds of events that cause unanticipated cardiac arrest. Such events initiate a frantic scramble for treatment, but clinicians spend the technical side of their careers preparing for sudden events. The cardiac arrests that almost always end poorly are the predictable ones.

A methodical, gradual approach to discussions about possible limits to medical treatment can work even when a person's health takes an unexpected turn. Hank was admitted to our ICU with pneumonia related to poor swallowing from a small stroke he sustained the year before. He could either be fed for the rest of his life by feeding tube, or he would ultimately die of a pneumonia caused by food and secretions falling into his lungs, what doctors call "aspiration." His daughter and

I scheduled a meeting to discuss future plans with Hank and his entire family for noon on the second day of his hospitalization. He was on some extra support for his breathing but had not yet required intubation.

Around 11 a.m. Hank was chatting pleasantly with his wife when he collapsed without warning from a dangerous heart rhythm called *torsades de pointes.* We resuscitated Hank and about ten days later liberated him from the ventilator. Having experienced life support firsthand, Hank decided that he didn't want intubation or cardiac resuscitation again. He felt confident that he was in life's final phase, and we and his family helped him wrap up his life. He died a month later, after he developed another pneumonia.

Critics might argue that we should have resolved Hank's "code status" the night before and therefore never treated his cardiac arrest. Our delay in discussing code status came at the price of more than a week on the ventilator. But instead of disappearing suddenly and wordlessly from the world, Hank left after a conscious period of wrapping up his life. In the brief window of time after his cardiac arrest, he was able to say farewell to his loved ones and put his affairs in order. Hank's apparent exception proves the rule that we can take time to be deliberate and reflective rather than immediately and reflexively deciding on a code status.

Meaningful "code status" discussions must focus on the person whose life is at stake—not just the procedures to be refused—and acknowledge uncertainty in a way that leaves room for both hope and realism.

The precise outcome of life-threatening illness is generally known only in retrospect. Any given ICU admission could end in a stunning save or a sad death. At times of great stress, it's easy to assume that the outcome has to be one way or the other. Premature certainty about outcome, often reflecting clinicians' biases, is part of why advance directives don't work. Patients and clinicians need a way to healthfully keep in mind all possible outcomes as they walk through the valley of shadows together. As I first struggled to explain what I meant, I found that families generally said that we were practicing how to "hope for the best" (meaningful survival and recovery) while "preparing for the worst" (an uncomfortable death). Preparing for the worst makes possible the conversion of a bad death to a better one.[7] This dual emphasis gives people room to consider hard questions in an overall context of hopefulness. And it lets them start thinking about what they might later regret, especially as it relates to finishing their lives.

Wrapping Up

Preparing for the worst means, in part, attending to life completion. The renowned palliative care physician Ira Byock has eloquently drawn on the writings of the psychologist Erik Erikson to describe the special tasks that matter near the end of life. The end of life, like its beginning and many middles, is a stage with activities and experiences particular to it. When we are lucky, we have the time to complete our lives by engaging in the tasks relevant to its last phases.[8] We can summarize, reconcile, bid farewell, provide counsel, and remember.

The completion tasks suited to life's end can occur throughout an ICU stay.[9] Normally used in hospice settings, Ira Byock's Four Things— "I love you," "Thank you," "Please forgive me," and "I forgive you"— represent an excellent script for making peace with death. Harvey Chochinov's dignity therapy, another technique used in hospice, is about summarizing one's life and taking leave. It commonly results in a written statement meant to reflect a person's life philosophy to the loved ones who will carry his memory. Patients are not always awake enough to tell stories, but when they can do so, they and their families find meaning in this process. I combine Byock's and Chochinov's ideas in my own practice, telling people about the Four Things and encouraging them to take oral histories when they can.

There will be some people who face death alone, individuals departing life whose social connections are used up, for whatever reason. Sometimes this has happened because of addiction or poor choices; sometimes it's just family circumstance. New rituals may be necessary to honor those solitary individuals, and medical and related professionals may have to step up to the plate when family is absent. These exceptions prove the rule that the dying process calls out for a community ready to carry the person forward.

In the ICU, life completion often must occur quickly. Just because it's challenging, though, does not mean it isn't worth the effort. Creating space for life completion will take time, careful attention, and extensive research. But some reform could begin quickly, even in the early stages.

Sometimes we only have an hour or two for life completion. When I was younger I wanted to know yes or no, "full code" or "DNR/DNI" (Do Not Resuscitate/Do Not Intubate). And then I either intubated or I didn't. I could only see the impending procedure, not its place in the patient's life. I still occasionally hear clinicians say, "We need to intubate you so you don't die. Is that okay?" I said the same thing when I was younger. The transition onto life support can be one of the most important moments of a person's life, and patients often receive the casual, technical indifference of an auto mechanic asking for approval to fix a busted carburetor.

I no longer rush reflexively to intubate patients who have worsening lung failure. I have them use a specialized mask ("CPAP" or "BiPAP") that looks like a fighter-pilot mask and actually derives from World War II technology that allowed high-altitude flight before the era of pressurized cockpits. This CPAP mask supports their breathing, and I sometimes prescribe a small dose of medication to calm nerves and ease the shortness of breath. These steps usually buy us a couple of hours.

Then we talk about what mechanical ventilation will feel like and how likely they are to recover from the lung failure. I talk specifically about the difficulties the ventilator presents for communication with loved ones and the chance that the patient will not awaken. I tell them that if they do not survive, I don't want to steal from them the opportunity to wrap up their lives, to say the things that matter to their loved ones. I have come to call this the "going off to war" talk.

As with war, before intubation people hope for the best and brace themselves against the worst, as they acknowledge what they mean to each other. If patients do not survive their time on life support, they and their families will still have been able to wish them well and bid farewell. In my experience, this talk also allows patients and families to prepare better for what may await them, regardless of the medical outcome.

The "going off to war" or "hope for the best, prepare for the worst" talks I have with patients and families before intubation represent a much broader phenomenon. We clinicians need to improve our awareness and management of clinical crossroads.

RECOGNIZE THE CROSSROADS

Particularly in the phase of life when an older person transitions into being a patient in failing health, certain medical decisions will cast a very long shadow over an individual's final stages of life. In some distressing instances, the decisions made in those circumstances can deform a life and a death in ways that the individual would never have wanted. Intubation, which can rob an individual of the ability to communicate with loved ones, is an obvious crossroads, but there are many others.[10]

My coworker tells a story about his father-in-law, Ray. An eighty-nine-year-old retired pediatrician living alone, Ray had harbored an infection of his foot for several months before his children discovered it and forced him to go to the hospital. Ray had been in reasonable health despite the diabetes that allowed the infection to set up in his foot. He had resisted treatment because he did not want to be hospitalized or undergo invasive procedures. Once he entered the hospital, events moved inexorably toward amputation of his infected foot.

Ray died, slowly and miserably, over the next six months. He never forgave his family for the decision to remove his leg rather than let him go peacefully. No one had raised the possibility that Ray might rationally have wanted to consider hospice care rather than surgery. The medical decision about amputation came too suddenly, too dramatically, for Ray's family to do anything but acquiesce. And there wasn't any person or system available to give voice to Ray's preference for a natural death in the face of his advanced diabetes. He was awake and communicating the whole time: No advance directive could possibly have applied in Ray's situation when it mattered.

Ray's experience, like that of many others, recalls Wendell Berry's deeply affecting story, "Fidelity." In it, Berry describes the end-of-life experience of an older Kentucky farmer named Burley Coulter. His family and friends, desperate to be of service, take Burley to a hospital when he falls ill, and then they struggle to undo what they have inadvertently done, when Coulter doesn't improve under the hospital's care. For some people, clinical crossroads come to seem in retrospect like the moment they entered the event horizon of a black hole. They are pulled irresistibly toward an uncomfortable and heavily medicalized death.

A system able to identify warning signs and communicate when a crossroads is near would be a great boon. Identifying such crux moments does not mean refusing medical treatment, although some people will certainly choose an earlier, natural death at a crossroads. It does mean making it possible for people to navigate crucial decisions well informed and able to understand not just the medical risks and benefits but also the personal implications of those decisions. Such guidance when it matters is far more important than a hypothetical list of theoretical treatments to refuse in the event of unconsciousness.

Ray's amputation was one of many possible crossroads. Pacemakers represent another common crossroads. I met Ella after a frightening experience at church. Ninety-four and still going strong, she fainted during a dull sermon and began to shake, as happens sometimes after a fainting episode. The paramedics gave her a large dose of sedative in case she'd had a seizure. In the ER, she was asleep because of the sedative, so they intubated her, a common but often inappropriate response in busy ERs.

Ella was transferred to our ICU, where we let the sedative wear off and removed the breathing tube. We could see that the wiring in her heart was failing, and a dangerously low heart rate had caused her to faint. I spoke with her about her values and priorities. I said that in her phase of life a pacemaker often represents a clinical crossroads, and she could choose which path to take. One path would be the medical approach, including the insertion of a pacemaker. Another path would be to acknowledge that these troubles with the wiring in her heart would likely be her final illness and to emphasize nonmedical approaches to life completion. She chose to refuse the pacemaker and to meet, instead, with a palliative care physician. She and her family were grateful for the opportunity to begin their explicit preparations for her death, which would likely come in a few weeks to months, while she received high quality hospice care.

Getting the tone and framing right for the identification of medical crossroads is fraught with the risk of error. It's critical not to abandon our elders or hasten their death merely because they are weaker than they once were. We shouldn't invoke the power of disability stigma as a way to persuade people to stop treatments against their better judgment. Decisions against aggressive medical treatment at a crossroads must represent what the individual truly desires when he is well and fully supported and allowed to explore what is authentic to him as a person. I'm not persuaded that focusing on societal costs is a productive way forward. I don't believe in quotas to decide who can or cannot have particular kinds of treatment. We haven't even figured out yet whether quotas would be necessary if medical treatments were carefully personalized, and arguments about rationing have a way of short-circuiting the meaningful conversations that might personalize care. Perhaps we will still need to talk about rationing medical care for older individuals after we have developed systems for meaningful, soulful engagement of patients and families in their final journeys, but I believe we should wait until those systems are in place. Today, though, we should be open, in a compassionate way, about the option of allowing a natural transition into life's final phases as part of informed consent discussions around procedures or surgeries at potential crossroads.[11] To put it simply, we oughtn't be saying "If you don't do this procedure you'll die," but perhaps something like, "Some people in this situation feel that their life is coming to its natural end and don't want medical procedures to interfere with that process. Others prefer even aggressive treatment in the hopes of getting more time. How do you feel?"

To date, very little research has investigated how to recognize crossroads, let alone how to tailor medical responses to the values and priorities of individual patients and their families at a given crossroads. But even without much new research, a modified advance directive could state simply, "If I'm ever in a situation where I could choose to undergo medical treatments or choose instead to allow a natural death for myself, please advise me and my family of this before we start the treatments." Many clinicians I know worry about bringing up hard topics, believing they have not been given permission and that it is presumptuous to assume that someone is ready to acknowledge that death is near. A clear permission slip to have difficult conversations might be just the ticket, something that would encourage conversations without precommitting to hypotheticals.

Recognizing a clinical crossroads can be difficult, because decisions are made prospectively but regretted retrospectively, after the outcome is already known. Just as a thoughtless disregard for the future can lead to bad decisions, retrospective remorse can color our thinking in extreme ways. It's common to later regret a decision that was perfectly appropriate at the time. We must be careful to avoid thinking as if decisions can be made in pure retrospect.[12]

Some cognitive psychologists recommend a technique that can help balance prospect and retrospect. Imagine, in a "prospective post-mortem," that your decision ended badly. Ask yourself why. What went wrong? What could have been done to avoid the undesired outcome? Such a thought experiment may improve our clarity of thinking about certain decisions. Rather than the autopsy metaphor, though, I prefer "anticipated retrospect," which works much the same way: Think through what you may come to regret about a decision you made at a crossroads and then make plans that can flexibly respond to those potential problems. It's important not to believe that every decision will lead to catastrophe: A life lived in fear is not the goal. But an approach to the future that acknowledges and balances the competing demands of prospect and retrospect is crucial to understanding how to proceed at a clinical crossroads.

Anticipated retrospect could, for example, allow people to think through whether a pacemaker is likely to deform a death or give more life. If I have a pacemaker now, will it interfere with my dying later? If it were to start interfering with a natural death, what could I do to facilitate a more appropriate transition? Katy Butler's thought-provoking 2010 essay in the *New York Times Magazine*, amplified in her book *Knocking on Heaven's Door*, argues that her father's pacemaker in anticipation of hernia surgery represented an unrecognized crossroads. Although the real trouble for her father came some years after the initial pacemaker, as he developed dementia from a series of strokes that finally led to his death, Butler came to regret the presence of the pacemaker—which the doctors refused to turn off, even when the request appeared to represent his authentic wishes—in her father's life. She contrasted her father's decision to have a pacemaker to her mother's later decision to refuse heart surgery for a worn-out valve. In Butler's account her father died badly, her mother well. Whether we agree with the specifics of Butler's assessment or not, it is absolutely true that American physicians often mismanage clinical crossroads.

The research isn't mature yet, but clinicians and patients should be collaboratively seeking markers that would indicate whether a candidate for a procedure—pacemaker, surgery, intubation—is entering an agonizing twilight like Butler's father did. Part of anticipated retrospect is contingency planning: When would a pacemaker get turned off? How would we know that we're entering life's final chapter? For some patients, it would help to meet with a geriatrician or palliative medicine specialist before deciding on a pacemaker. Many pacemakers would still be placed, but some would not. That contingency planning is part of what's missing from most advance directives because they are so focused on procedures in generic, hypothetical circumstances rather than events likely to happen to the given individual, along with the later eventualities.

In any case—and this is a point that cardiologists are finally coming around to and palliative care physicians have long embraced—it's appropriate to turn off a pacemaker or equivalent device when the time comes.[13] This would take some careful planning and preparation and the allowance that it might lead to death within a few minutes or not for several months, but in the right circumstance, clinicians should be prepared to honor requests to stop a cardiac device. Such a decision shouldn't be undertaken lightly, but it can be a healthful part of the transition to hospice and the embrace of life's end.

As part of identifying and communicating clinical crossroads, we should be tying advance care planning to what actually lies ahead for individual patients. To create relevant guidance requires knowing something about the expected course of a given illness, not the standard list of hypothetical events. A guide should have a map of the route they will be taking up the mountain. To expect advance directives to work without bonding them to actual decisions and an expected course is naïve and ultimately confusing.[14]

In a collaboration with a group of researchers at Boston University, we evaluated one hundred thousand outpatients over the age of sixty-five, to see how many of them would end up in an ICU on a ventilator within five years. We developed and tested a numeric score, based on the medical conditions they had at the time of their first visit. We found that a small handful of risk factors, including diabetes, high blood pressure, and emphysema, could be used to divide individuals into low, moderate, and high risk groups. The large majority of these individuals were in the low risk category.[15] Our score was, to the best of our knowledge, the first attempt to create such a predictive score that could help people make concrete plans for their immediate futures. (Other researchers had used a simple age cutoff to suggest when advance care planning should begin. Our findings suggest that this approach was too pessimistic about age, sending a message of "Welcome to retirement; prepare to die," rather than "How can we best prepare for medical events you may soon encounter?"[16])

Predictive tools could also be used for counseling, preparation for rehabilitation, or enrollment in special studies of new treatment options. Prediction models could be used to help tailor rehabilitation and support plans that could be much more flexible than contracts, able to accommodate the inevitable changes in status that occur. In some circumstances, predictions could help people to prepare for the worst while hoping for the best.

None of these approaches will work in a vacuum: Community and companionship will be central to durable solutions.

CREATE A SUPPORT COMMUNITY

Patients and families will be better able to identify clinical crossroads if they have communities to support them in the effort. Careful attention to the building and maintenance of communities is especially important. Two expansions of community make sense right away. We've already seen that families need a place at the table in terms of PFACs and open visitation. New experts of several different kinds may also prove important in spanning the gap between clinicians and patients/families. Guidance will be a team effort that includes more than just traditional clinicians.

Chaplains, where they exist, may be helpful—they receive excellent training and have a proven track record of caring for people of various faiths, including strict atheists. While they've fallen out of favor in the increasingly commercial environment of American medicine, hospital chaplains have expertise that allows them to respond to people's human needs in the midst of a crisis. With some focused education on supporting people through shared decision making during life-threatening illness, hospital chaplains could become central again to the proper function of a hospital.[17]

In some hospitals, social workers have filled the role of chaplains, although financial pressures often force social workers to focus on negotiations with insurance companies and other healthcare facilities. Some hospitals have created positions for palliative care nurses or communication specialists to assist people in the navigation of serious illness. Bud Hammes's group in Wisconsin hired advance care planning specialists, and the availability of these professionals was vital to the successes in La Crosse.

The trusted guides who are increasingly part of the teams helping women navigate childbirth may offer lessons for the ICU. Childbirth, like dying, is a natural experience that was medicalized in the twentieth century. But the pendulum is swinging back as more women are now giving birth at home and are involving nonmedical guides, such as midwives and sometimes "doulas." Doulas, from the Greek word for household servants, are trained to accompany women during the experience of giving birth.[18] An experienced navigator, or "sickbed doula," who is not a medical professional may be perfect company in the valley of shadows.[19]

By sickbed doula, I don't mean hospice workers, although professionals in palliative care may well provide the services of a sickbed doula in some communities. Hospice has historically worked when everyone has agreed that death is near. But when death *may* be near, the system does a terrible job of structuring environments in which people can flourish. The role of the sickbed doula would not be medical, but supportive and interpretive, helping patients and families understand what is at stake as decisions arise during the ICU admission and helping them navigate the immense psychological distress that many encounter.

Such doulas or non-clinician guides could mediate between the technical proficiency of the physician and the moral sensibilities of patients, helping the two groups to understand each other. Family members who have been through an ICU admission with a loved one could be ideal sickbed doulas for future patients and families.

Sickbed doulas might allow, for patients whose time proves to be near its end, for the return of some rituals for the deathbed. Simplified rituals, not necessarily religious, could mark impending death and honor the final phase of a person's life.[20] In today's technology-laden ICU there rarely is time or opportunity for such observances. But until there are possibilities for meaning at the end of life, all that remains for physicians and families is to perceive death as failure. I served as a doula for my friend Jeff Valentine shortly before his death from myeloma. It is one of the treasured memories of my life.

Where a patient has a strong attachment to a specific religious community, traditional clergy could function as sickbed doulas. Even where hospital chaplains have been available, medical professionals have often kept individuals' personal ministers at arm's length. Because these tasks have not, in this form and with this rigor, been a part of their duties before, denominational clergy would require additional training to improve their ability to elicit patients' values and help with the identification of clinical crossroads. Hospital chaplaincy programs, departments of social work, and new curricula could easily be made available within religious communities to help to expand and personalize their work as sickbed doulas for individuals within their communities.

New voices and new perspectives will help to change assumptions about how and why medical technology might be used.

CREATE SPACE FOR FACILITATED FAREWELLS

Linda was a slender brunette in her midforties who was dying of amyotrophic lateral sclerosis, or ALS. Once known as Lou Gehrig's disease, ALS slowly paralyzes its victims, who generally die of lung failure. Linda was at home, on hospice, when she broke her upper arm during a transfer out of bed, and she ended up in the ER for an entire day as emergency doctors tried to figure out what to do with her. During her first months on hospice, she'd needed only occasional support from the hospice nurse, but while her fractured arm just needed a splint, she couldn't care for herself at home any more. After twenty agonizing hours in the ER she developed low blood oxygen levels, and the ER doctor asked me to admit her to the ICU for respiratory failure, too embarrassed to tell me that she was already on hospice because we don't usually admit patients from hospice to the ICU.

As I began to discuss with Linda the events of the last day, I was glad that we had ignored the usual practice of excluding hospice patients from the ICU. Despite hospice, Linda hadn't quite realized that she was in the process of dying, and she acknowledged to me that her children were even less aware of how little time she had left. We made calls and pestered the airlines to allow her children to come to her bedside. Linda and I discussed the documents that categorically refused life support technologies and ICU admission. I proposed to her that we use a semi-invasive lung support system to allow her to stay alive long enough to see her children one last time. She looked deeply relieved as she agreed with the plan.

As horrifying as it was for an elegant woman barely into middle age to be facing death, her transfer to the ICU allowed crucial time for Linda and her children to gather, to process her imminent death, and to complete their lives together. If we had applied a simple interpretation of her living will and her associated decision to enter hospice, we never would have accepted Linda into the ICU. Why spend medical resources to prolong a patient's life for a day or two? Linda and her family would have thereby lost their chance to say goodbye. That would have been a tragedy.

I believe firmly that advanced medical care has a place beyond merely resisting death. In specific settings, it is appropriate to provide even "futile" life support. One victim of drowning was terribly ill on the ventilator and not obviously improving. She was DNR/DNI but had been intubated by paramedics during the frantic minutes beside the lake where she drowned. In part we wanted to wait long enough to see whether she would improve rapidly as some patients do, even though recovery was very unlikely. More importantly, though, her son was serving in the military and was slowly wending his way to her bedside on military transports. Once he arrived, the family gathered and allowed her to finish the natural process of dying.

I believe that facilitated farewell also occurs when we give families time to come to terms with tragedy. One woman came to our ICU nearly dead after a fall at her nursing home. We spent the better part of a day attempting resuscitation while her family came to terms with her death. Such treatments shouldn't override sincere, informed rejections of further treatment, and they must not inflict suffering on the patient, but sometimes life support can reassure families that there was an attempt made to meaningfully forestall death. Such reassurance can give frightened families some time to move from utter shock to appropriate behaviors in anticipation of death.

Sometimes a well-supported farewell requires that a clinician accept a nurturing rather than a technical role. I remember Sven, a man slowly dying of advanced heart failure who had developed significant internal bleeding that was cutting off circulation to his abdominal organs. We scheduled him for urgent surgery, but his heart stopped before we could get him to the operating room. We performed aggressive CPR with Sven's family in the room. We even attempted an emergency surgery in the ICU room in an attempt to bring him back, but ultimately we could make no progress.

Sven's wife and children wept at his bedside, and I felt the stress of being divided between consoling them and working toward Sven's recovery. Nonetheless, research suggests that families do better when they see CPR—and in my experience there's always some clinician who can guide them through the experience as the frantic procedure occurs, so I attended to them, holding my arm over his wife's shoulder and explaining what we were doing.[21]

After a death, the images from last days, weeks, or months of life may be what stay longest with grieving families. For all the rhetoric about how important it is to humanize people's last days, policy makers and clinicians often fail to see ways that even ICU care could help people finish their lives with the people they love.

Matt, a researcher friend, once asked me to review a survey he was administering to American physicians. Trying to understand inappropriate use of ICU resources, he created an ICU admission scenario that seemed obviously futile to him. He chose a patient with cancer and six months left to live, coming to the ICU with a serious bacterial infection. Matt expected that all physicians would agree that this was a case where the ICU should not be used. (Such is the practice in Australia or Britain, where critical care resources are more limited than in the United States.) What Matt saw as absolutely clear was missing crucial information, though. "Has the patient completed his life yet?" I asked. Six months can be a span of life worth fighting for if it can create an opportunity for life completion and taking leave of loved ones. Depending on the specific circumstances of an individual life, Matt's extreme scenario might have been entirely appropriate for the ICU, as part of a facilitated farewell. The discussion with Matt reminded me how much of the problems we confront in the ICU arise from failures of clinicians to see the world the way their patients do.

CHANGE THE FRAMING TO MANAGE CLINICIANS' MORAL DISTRESS

Laypeople may not understand how painful it is for many clinicians to perform CPR or administer life support to a person with a high risk of death. This intense moral distress is part of what has led to the current approach to advance care planning. Since clinician moral distress plays such a significant role in the failings of advance directives, it's important to tackle that distress head on.

I have seen moral distress affect even technical procedures. While the "slow code" of yesteryear (in which clinicians "walk, don't run" to the patient's room, thereby only pretending to perform CPR) is no longer openly practiced, I still see lackadaisical CPR performed. Beyond the dishonesty inherent in such charades, there's the risk that clinicians will reinforce sloppy technique. High-quality CPR requires extensive practice, which can be corrupted if some CPR attempts are half-hearted. When it matters, clinicians may be less able to perform good CPR. The framing I now use with other clinicians is that they are doing two things when they provide professional, high-quality CPR (assuming CPR does not violate the patient's wishes). First, they are participating in a distinctly American ritual related to mortality that many individuals value as a protest against the inevitability of death. Second, they are maintaining CPR skills that will allow them—when time is of the essence—to use CPR in ways that give people a significant opportunity for meaningful, high-quality life. Remember that CPR is among the most successful of medical procedures as judged by the "number needed to treat."

As deathbed rituals go, CPR is not the strangest in human history. It can be a reasonable way to shake our fists against the sky. Dogmatic claims about whether and when CPR can be performed miss the point entirely. Even unsuccessful CPR is not morally wrong unless it deforms death or violates a person's values and priorities. In my experience, stressing the interdependence of all patients who receive CPR and the ritual aspects of the procedure ameliorates some of the moral distress clinicians feel. Again, my point is to be sure that CPR is well tailored to the individual patient, and it's the individual's characteristics rather than clinicians' dislike for CPR that should matter most.

CHANGING CULTURE OUTSIDE MEDICINE

Interdependence and cultural messages matter outside the ICU as well. *Media vita in morte sumus* is a phrase that has circulated among Christians for many centuries: "In the midst of life we are in death." No one knows who first said those words. In America we know the statement best from the Anglican Book of Common Prayer, as part of the guidebook for many Protestant funerals, but the phrase arose long before the Reformation. Most believe that the language comes from an old French hymn, perhaps as early as the eighth century. Whatever the source of this saying, it contains centuries of wisdom. Independent of its Christian origin, we in contemporary society have lost track of the phrase and its power. And that is a serious problem.

On one reading of the phrase, it is less true now than when it entered the world. While it is still true that death could come at any moment—a heart attack, a car accident, or a blood clot to the lungs—it is statistically true that our death in any given year of our lives is improbable. People do not all suddenly die of cholera or typhoid fever or plague anymore. Sore throat isn't necessarily diphtheria or the desperately fatal "black canker"; it's just a nuisance virus or maybe a touch of Strep that is easily treated with amoxicillin. From that medical and epidemiological perspective, in the midst of life we are less in death than any prior period of human history. Of course when death does strike, especially when it comes early or unexpectedly, we struggle to understand where the time has gone. Because no matter how much later we now die than humans used to, we still all die.

It's been easy to see prior death culture as irrelevant because of the epidemiological changes that separate the present from the past. Their culture may seem relevant only when premature death is rampant. But our ancestors were not making a simple actuarial statement about the causes and timing of death. They weren't just saying, "Infectious diseases and trauma are killing us at staggering rates. We should build a religion to deal with it." They were only half talking about the timing of death when they referred to death "in the midst of life." They were also making a normative statement about life.

Living in the midst of death is about the exquisite clarity that comes from knowing that life is temporary. Conventional wisdom says that life flashes before your eyes when you come to die, but that's not really been the experience I've witnessed in my patients. It's more that various old, persistent memories percolate to the top, much as you see in a person with advancing dementia who remembers every detail of life from forty years ago but none from forty minutes ago. But there is important truth in the idea of a life's meaning becoming visible when death beckons. Death brings into sharp focus what we have meant by our lives. Even if it's not true of the deathbed proper, the specter of death can help most of us conceive our entire lives anew.

We are mortal. We will die. But we humans are like nothing else in the universe; we are conscious beings. And when we come to die, the truth of our mortality can come crashing down on us. But the irruption of that truth into awareness can shape our lives in compelling ways. That is the point of the old Christian phrase. There is deep and beautiful life to be had in the acknowledgment of mortality.

There is no question that contemporary culture makes it difficult to acknowledge death. Changing that will take time and coordinated effort. We can and should acknowledge that life is fleeting and that much of its beauty resides in that transience. By acknowledging that we will one day die, we can intensify our relationships while we live. Allowing such an acknowledgement will make it easier to confront the possible end of life in the setting of an ICU admission. I'm aware of the heartfelt and valid concerns like those raised by the writer Susan Sontag and her son David Rieff.[22] The two of them felt that human mortality could only ever be a sick joke, and attempts to find meaning in the face of death were only so much petty delusion. Many people would I suspect agree with them. Some of us will never be able to come to terms with our own passage from life.

Whether we ever make peace with the reality of death or rage against it until the bitter end, living with awareness of death has certain practical implications.

The most common regret I hear as an ICU physician, other than family members' sadness at a loved one's passing, is that they wish they had said certain things when that person was still alive. Too many things are routinely left unsaid. In large part that's because we feel with special intensity when we confront death. But we can communicate with each other deeply before death comes.

A much-simplified version of the old Christian phrase says to "Live every day as if it were your last." That's a complicated saying too. It seems to suggest that we should not waste a single day, that we should savor the beauty life has to offer with all the vigor we can muster. It might also suggest that we should do great things we would otherwise procrastinate away. The concept of a "bucket list" is based on that concept. While I support living life to its fullest and recognize that the specter of death motivates a certain immediacy in experiencing rare or special things, I am skeptical of a bucket list of adventures as a response to mortality. It's not that we shouldn't dream and achieve, but there is much more to life than a list of expensive vacations or risky spectacles.

Living life in the midst of death means creating relationships in the presence of our confounding temporariness. It means recognizing that we will grow and age and sometimes lose our way. Life in the presence of death means consistently treating people with the marvelous, tender poignancy that arises spontaneously when we discover that they might die. Death helps us to emphasize the ideal over the actual and to do so in a way that moves reality closer to that ideal.

The Simpsons grappled with these questions in 1991, in an episode ("One Fish, Two Fish, Blowfish, Blue Fish") in which Homer, the father of the famously dysfunctional cartoon family, eats Japanese blowfish that has been improperly prepared. (Always ravenous, he eats the prized and dangerous delicacy the way most people eat potato chips.) When the chef's mistake is revealed, Homer becomes certain that he has ingested a fatal dose of Fugu toxin and spends the evening making peace with his loved ones. After a hectic night, he discovers, when the sun rises, that he had not in fact been poisoned. True to form, he immediately settles back into a meaningless existence of junk food and television. But the magic of that day stays with us as viewers. We do not want to live every day the way Homer lived his, rushing frantically to cross items off his bucket list, but we want the clarity of vision that Homer experienced during what he thought was his last day.

As my wife and I lived through her cancer diagnosis and the surgery to remove her eye, we felt both the dread and the strength associated with the reality that we will someday die. Whether the end comes by cancer or heart disease or a car crash, we cannot negotiate our way out of our final mortality. Her eye cancer forced us to acknowledge that fact. Our relationship has deepened, and we have been able to find what is sacred and meaningful in the shadow of death. These meanings are quite independent of the medical system. Such clear vision of a more substantial and intimate life may also contribute to better care in the ICU, as culture and medicine work together.

NOT LEFT UNSAID

One thing advance care planning gets right is that it's better not to wait until it is too late to say or do certain things. In the rush of life, we commonly forget to acknowledge how important we are to each other. Unusual events or crises are usually required to make such emotional conversations possible, but by then it may be too late. In my own struggle to find a balance between forgetfulness and awkwardness, I've settled on writing letters to the people I love. I call these my "Not Left Unsaid" letters, and they contain what I want to be sure I have told them before one of us dies. I want to know that I've said how much I love them and why. To be sure that I have forgiven and sought forgiveness where that is needed.

With a nice pen on fine paper, I now write letters to people who matter to me. Not every year, but often enough to maintain rich relationships. I have used Thanksgiving and birthdays as the time for these letters. Thanksgiving has the advantage of already providing a natural context for "giving of thanks." For religious people Easter or Yom Kippur might work even better. It's helpful to have some sort of deadline, but what matters most is just writing the letters.

I write the letters to be read right away, not as posthumous epistles. It is a slow process, and the letters don't always say precisely what I want them to. That's the nature of language. My loved ones have been patient with the inadequacies of human communication: These letters have become moments of precious connection. I began by using Ira Byock's Four Things[23] as a way to structure these Not Left Unsaid letters, and my practice has evolved from there.

I've learned some things along the way. A letter seems to be easier than an oral conversation, at least for me. Letters can be stored and retrieved, and many people will find it easier to be honest and tender in a letter. Electronic mail is too informal, too ephemeral, so I write them out longhand. Also, this kind of communication should be private. People don't like hypocrites or show-offs, and they will sense when such a letter isn't really for their benefit. Along those lines, I mostly ask for forgiveness and tell people what I like most about them. This practice has a way of clarifying my vision and theirs.

While part of life completion is summarizing the meaning of an individual life, I try to resist the temptation to preach sermons about the good life. I include one or two elements of what I treasure, but I don't want my letters to leave recipients imagining Benjamin Franklin yammering on about personal accountability and waking up before sunrise. In my experience people want to be loved, engaged, forgiven, and asked for forgiveness. With rare exceptions, they do not want to sit through a sanctimonious lecture. I expect that when I come closer to my time to die I will engage in something like Chochinov's dignity therapy with a formal statement of my life's philosophy. For now, I'm sticking with the basics.

I suspect that communication will be easier when crisis comes if it is not the first time that we have spoken to each other deeply and authentically, aware of our mortality. Occasional discussion about values and priorities relevant to medical care when death may be near make the most sense in the human context of meaningful conversations. The medical details are not, in my view, what matter most. But the discussions triggered by Not Left Unsaid letters could very easily catalyze the kinds of discussions that could replace advance directives.

Most or all of us want to find some kind of meaning in the fact of our death. That is difficult but possible; these Not Left Unsaid letters can help. Simultaneously, we all should seek to find meaning in the dying. As a society we ought to find ways to feel more comfortable learning from the dying, serving them, and spending time in their presence. Too often when we think of the dying, we think of wasted medical resources rather than opportunities for learning and transformation. We should be volunteering to take meals to the dying or disabled, sitting with them, and hearing what they have to say. As Atul Gawande so eloquently advocated in his *Being Mortal*, we have a societal duty to reform nursing homes and similar environments so that people can flourish there.[24] Such work will stretch us beyond what is comfortable, but it's effort better spent than the channeling of disability stigma within the current system.

AUTHENTIC PERSONALIZATION

Treating the experience of life-threatening illness as if it were a problem for a contract to avoid medical care has contributed to the failures of advance directives. This framing has driven the questions asked and answered most often: "When can physicians override your family's desire to keep you alive?" or "Should we ever perform CPR?" But these aren't the most important questions. To get personalization right will require asking different questions.

Our group at Intermountain prefers to think of advance care planning in terms of Personalized Care during Serious Illness. From this perspective, the better questions to ask include "What phase of life are you living in now?" "How do you like information to be presented to you?" "Would it *ever* be okay with you if your family and/or your physicians decided that further medical technology wasn't of service to you?" "Are there any specific things that you worry about if you were to develop a serious illness?" These questions will also need to start getting at the problems of how people view agency and autonomy in medical decision making.

The one question that current advance directives get right is "Who are the people that matter most to you?" but that question gets asked in a limited way: a name, phone number and address and, perhaps, whether they can override the instructions in the attached living will. But it matters a great deal whether those people are well supported in their efforts to speak for you. For this support to be useful, clinicians need to know something about those family members. How do they process information? Have they thought about what it might mean to allow a natural death? What frightens them about the experience of speaking for a loved one in the ICU? What are their emotional vulnerabilities and blind spots? Real solutions will have to start asking those questions.

Good questions are a start, but answers matter too. People generally do not know what they want. They have deep and strongly held preferences, but those preferences are not captured by living wills. Without extensive education and experience, most people don't know how to map their own values and priorities onto specific medical decisions. This step will be crucial to solving the problems with advance directives.

The adaptive, computerized advance directive, Making Your Wishes Known, while still preliminary, is the furthest along of any current efforts to tailor recommendations to people's actual preferences. Much more research will be required to understand how decisions are made and experienced. Individuals have different personality types, information-processing styles, social support networks, and susceptibility to psychological distress. They are living at different phases of life. These aspects of their personalities matter and are simply not addressed with contemporary advance directives.

While more research is required, certain strategies—specialized games, values elicitation procedures, and guided reflections—have shown promise. I expect and hope that we will test and adopt sophisticated methods for helping people decide what their own values and priorities are and how they relate to decisions about medical treatments. It's not enough to have people check off boxes on a legal form. We should be using all our wits to understand best how to serve people in their actual individuality.

The problems in current medical practice are about more than decisions. They're also about how people experience medical crisis and life-threatening illness. Personalities and vulnerabilities and life histories matter not just for guiding medical decisions, but also for what is suffered and hungered after in the valley of shadows. Even when no decision is ever made, patients and families deserve tailored supports. The research to define who's at risk and how best to sustain them during a crisis is quite early, but it's promising and needs to be continued. Independent of these necessary improvements in personalization, more relevant categories of decisions could help.

A POSSIBLE MAP: FIVE APPROACHES TO INTENSIVE CARE

Whatever replaces advance directives should include a better approach to decision architecture. The goal should be an architecture that is personally relevant and aims to align the actions taken by the medical system (which includes decisions by patients, families, and clinicians) with the patient's actual values, goals, and priorities.[25] It will also need to acknowledge the fact that for many people the question of medical care relates more than anything to their phase of life before the critical illness.

As I have walked with many hundreds of people through the valley of shadows over the years, I've noticed that their goals and sensibilities tend to fall into several basic approaches to questions of how aggressively to pursue medical treatments when life is threatened.

A reasonably simple schema could employ five categories, clustered roughly around typical goals and the decisions associated with them.

Such a system would acknowledge that sometimes CPR is the right thing and sometimes it's the wrong thing to do, even in a single person's life at a particular moment in time.

In this section I lay out the five basic approaches that in my experience people prefer. Each approach encapsulates a given philosophy about the balance between risks and benefits of aggressive medical treatment, tied to the goals those treatments can achieve.[26] Most people will change their preferred approach based on their life philosophy and phase of life, but at any given time healthcare workers could be directed by a given approach toward patient-relevant goals.

Approach 1: Do Everything

For decades "do everything" has been the best-known response to life-threatening illness. It is still the strategy most consistent with many Americans' sensibilities about terminal illness. For many otherwise healthy people, this seems appropriate. Such individuals have a higher likelihood of responding to treatments, however heroic, and the sense of tragedy if they were to die is sufficiently greater than the risk of a deformed death to make "do everything" the appropriate line of attack. This is the approach of many young parents. Although I recognize the risks of discomfort and expense associated with this approach, I want to pursue it while my own children are young. In most respects, this overlaps with the traditional "full code" designation. On this model, clinicians should do anything and everything they can to prolong life.

Unfortunately, in many cases this default setting may not be the right response to life-threatening illness. It has probably been overused in individuals with advanced terminal diseases, at the extremes of age, or with permanent loss of consciousness. Because the debates about permanent vegetative state are so contentious, it may be reasonable to specify separately an Approach 1 that endorses treatment in a confirmed permanent vegetative state versus an Approach 1 that refuses treatment in such a condition. (Evidence suggests that only a small minority of Americans want to be kept alive in a permanent vegetative state; I certainly do not. Recall that this is an exceedingly rare situation regardless.)

Honest, open discussion is crucial, even when something like Approach 1 is chosen. This approach to life-threatening illness must not be used to rob people of opportunities to complete their lives. They should hope for the best but prepare for the worst. Choosing this approach requires deep commitment to excellent rehabilitation after life-threatening illness to help minimize the symptoms of Post Intensive Care Syndrome and to help people flourish in the face of new disability. It is morally wrong to agree to run life support technologies and then abandon patients to their own devices once they have made it out of the ICU alive. Even this most aggressive and familiar approach cannot continue in the dehumanizing currents of the past.

Approach 2: Be Aggressive Only if I Have a Reasonable Chance of Recovery

If one takes the more common serious medical conditions requiring ICU admission (septic shock and severe lung injury, for instance) and considers them together, about 70–75 percent of patients will survive the hospitalization. Overall about half of survivors of critical illnesses like those will suffer both psychological and physical disability afterward. That means that on average something like 30 to 40 percent of patients admitted to ICUs with substantial critical illness will ultimately have a strongly positive recovery and another 30 percent will have Post Intensive Care Syndrome, within which they will be able to thrive, albeit on new terms. Recovery will cost them a great deal in terms of their pain and discomfort during the hospitalization, especially during the ICU stay, but by about six to twelve months after hospitalization these survivors will often have a reasonable to excellent quality of life.

Where Approach 1 is the extreme package, Approach 2 would be something like a standard package: Use aggressive medical treatments as long as the chances of recovery are reasonable.

Many people who have reached maturity without substantial illness or disability will consider this approach as most relevant to their situation. Because they have lived reasonably healthy lives, they have a greater probability of recovering and they have not yet reached a stage where they feel that life is near its end. Importantly, they have also lived to maturity, and the sting of death may have lost some of its power because they have seen their children reach adulthood, or have achieved what they will in their careers. They have had what seems to them a full life, even if they would like another couple decades to enjoy it.

My proposed cutoff seems reasonable for two reasons. First, the chance of survival is high enough that I think most people who are not yet ready to depart life would be willing to undergo the discomfort, confusion, and pain that is associated with substantial intensive care. Second, it represents the average ICU course for people with acute, severe illness. The average seems worth defending even if the therapies we use to defend it are uncomfortable. While we were committed to Approach 1—do whatever it takes, even when the chances of survival are less than 10 percent—for Kristi, the young mother with a terrible Strep infection, she only ever became sick enough that Approach 2 was relevant to guide her treatment. Her degree of illness, however startling, was par for the course in a contemporary ICU, and most patients survive it well.

Approach 2 requires more consideration of the individual's trajectory. It acknowledges that in some circumstances it might be better to allow a natural death rather than continue with medical treatments that are unlikely to succeed. When a patient's course begins to deviate from the expected average course, discussions about a natural death should arise. Most life support technologies would be routinely applied in most patients. Cardiopulmonary resuscitation would be performed for reversible causes but would not be used for typically irreversible causes. If CPR did not result in recovery of consciousness, clinicians would promptly transition to allowing a natural death to occur.

Approach 3: Only Admit Me to the Intensive Care Unit if I Have an Excellent Chance of Recovery

The idea behind Approach 3 is that life is close to wrapping up but sudden death is not yet welcome. Aggressive medical treatment—with its attendant pain, expense, and discomfort—would make sense only if there were excellent chances of recovery. I find an increasing number of patients with chronic medical conditions favoring something like this when they come under my care. An ICU stay for a bleeding ulcer would make sense, even if it involved temporary intubation, because the large majority of patients do quite well after such an episode. For severe pneumonia, on the other hand, someone who adopted Approach 3 would probably not undergo mechanical ventilation because, while many patients do recover well, the odds of recovery are not "excellent." Most people would not want CPR unless it were for a witnessed, easily resuscitated problem, such as might happen with an unexpected, transient heart rhythm problem. Approach 3 would generally apply to people who are just beginning the final phases of life and do not yet see their lives as complete. They might find their current health manageable but acknowledge that further decreases in strength and quality of life would probably cross a threshold for them that would indicate that their life is near its end.

I'm aware that there will be some difficulties with honoring the precise spirit of this request, particularly with current holes in medical understanding. More research is required to understand what "excellent chances" might mean and how commonly various diagnoses are associated with those outcomes. But that is achievable with focused research. Patients choosing this approach would commonly be encouraged to attend to life completion tasks even though they may have several years of reasonable quality of life, assuming that they do not develop a new, serious illness. People in this relatively gray zone would want and need extra supports to help them navigate their decisions and the implications. It might be a geriatrician or a palliative medicine doctor in the outpatient arena and a sickbed doula on the inpatient side who provide that guidance. These preparations wouldn't be intended to persuade them not to waste medical resources, but to help them live their lives more fully, even when death may be near. These are people who would be ideal candidates for the slow medicine approach.[27]

Approach 4: Don't Admit Me to the Intensive Care Unit

Within Approach 4, the ICU serves as a marker of a disease process that will cause significant suffering and discomfort, with only modest probabilities of recovery. For many individuals, particularly those late in life or after protracted chronic illness, this approach will be appealing. On this view a mild urinary infection, one that could be tackled with antibiotics and fluids on a normal hospital ward, would be reasonable to treat. Treating such simple diseases would not deform the process of dying, or substitute a peaceful and relatively pain-free death for a more arduous and uncomfortable death shortly thereafter. But a disease severe enough that the individual would likely die without ICU admission would be the signal that a natural death was underway. In that event, medical professionals would encourage a good death by supporting life completion while strengthening individuals' communities. In settings like this, a sickbed doula or palliative care nurse might leave the ICU and come out to a regular hospital ward for consultation and support.

This approach does not make sense for people actively in the process of dying, who generally would adopt Approach 5. I anticipate that I will prefer Approach 4 in my later seventies or if I have a serious chronic illness, although I know that I will reassess these questions periodically as I experience maturity and illness. The urgency of correct, useful information about prognosis is no less pressing here than in the other approaches. To make room for the community of a healthful deathbed, loved ones must know when the end is near.

Clinicians must not be afraid to speak honestly about the transitions they are observing in a body's function and the medical aspects of the phase of life. Even when ICU admission is not desired, communicating that death appears imminent is crucial to allow participants to play their roles in life completion. I believe that my grandfather Howard would have chosen Approach 4. Had this approach been explicitly described and endorsed, his team may have known to tell us about his situation and allowed us to say goodbye.

Approach 5: Don't Admit Me to a Hospital; Focus Only on My Comfort

This final approach indicates that the person has reached the point in her life when artificially prolonging life no longer seems appropriate under any circumstances. This would be the approach when medicine promises only or primarily deformation of the experience of dying. This would overlap substantially with hospice care as it is currently employed. In the past, this approach has been mostly reserved for patients with advanced cancer, after the "failure" of chemotherapy. We must recognize that more diseases than cancer could justify such a belief that biomedical treatments aimed at postponing death are no longer welcome in a person's life.

Approach 5 emphasizes that there is a difference between the actual primary burden or discomfort associated with a treatment and the burden or discomfort that results from postponing death. Antibiotics are a classic example. By and large (assuming you don't get diarrhea or a rash), antibiotics are not associated with any particular discomfort. But over the course of human history, worn-out bodies have tended to die from urinary tract infection or pneumonia. These conditions, if the symptoms are managed well, can be peaceful ways to pass from life. However, these infections are also pretty easy to cure, and it's difficult to resist the temptation to treat them. Antibiotics aren't uncomfortable, and the cure rate for each episode is high. But in the process, treatment may substitute a more painful death a short time later. The risk is not that the antibiotic treatment will be painful or directly burdensome. The risk is also not only that death will be delayed or more expensive. The real risk, and the one we should be careful of, is that the treatment will deform the process of dying.[28] Approach 5 acknowledges that the purpose of medicine is no longer to cure disease but to maintain comfort in life's final phase.

My Five Approaches represent an imperfect map. This simple schema will require research to make it useful, and helping people choose their Approach—and adjusting their choice as life conditions change—will not solve all the problems of living wills. People will need cues to understand how to map their own goals, priorities, and aspirations onto even these Five Approaches. Insights from psychology and choice architecture will help in this process. For most people, this is a question of how they perceive their phase of life. We need to understand better how this process works in modern society and the era of extreme autonomy. The traditional laser-sharp focus on procedures represents the interests of doctors and lawyers but not, in general, patients and families. An advantage to these Five Approaches is that they focus on patient-relevant outcomes and the contexts of care that are relevant to the phases of life in which they are most likely to apply.

Clinicians will need clear instructions about how to map a given patient's status onto hospital "code" protocols. The usual infrastructure for codes will need to evolve, if it is going to be truly patient-centered, to distinguish between recoverable and nonrecoverable forms of cardiac arrest. With a little patience and research, such methods could be perfected and implemented. An advantage to the Five Approaches is that it could allow stable integration into code protocols.

A hypothetical case may suggest what a personalized ICU experience might look like. Joan is a seventy-two-year-old woman with long-standing diabetes who is admitted to the ICU with a severe pneumonia. When she arrives in the ICU, she is supported with a noninvasive pressure mask and assigned a doula, who helps her and her husband think through several questions about their communication approach (once a day, with the doula present), their preferences for information (all information, positive or negative, not holding any punches), and their sense about what phase of life Joan is in (has lived well; would not yet see death as a release). On the basis of these conversations, her physicians propose Approach 2 and ask her whether it accurately represents her wishes. She agrees and comments that if she suffered a cardiac arrest, she will want natural death if she hasn't clearly awakened by the third day after CPR, and she thinks seven days on the ventilator is the maximum time she would be willing to spend unless she was clearly improving on day 7. Her doula, her family, and her medical team all remember the conversation and make a record of it in the chart.

A day later, her lungs worsen to the point that the pressure mask is no longer sufficient, so after her family hugs and kisses her as part of a "going off to war" talk, she is intubated. On the ventilator, the team keeps her off sedation so that she can interact using an eye-tracking tablet computer, and by the third day on the ventilator she is walking around the ICU, albeit hesitantly and with substantial assistance. She is extubated on day 8 and takes about two months to get home. From there, an Aftercare and Recovery Center helps her make her way through the eight months it takes to get back to about 70 percent of her prior strength. While she wishes desperately that she had never fallen ill, she has made peace with her new physical limitations and is glad to be alive.

Although Joan's case is idealized, something like her experience is almost possible in a small number of ICUs today; we should be working to make it a reality in every modern ICU.

I've described a vision for how the ICU can change in the near future. I have talked about the problems with the current system, and they are many. But I don't favor pessimism. There is momentum within society and the medical community for real and substantial change. There's much to look forward to. A humane ICU, brimming with healing and meaning, is within our reach.

What Should We Do
in the Meanwhile?

In this book I've laid out a sustained criticism of the way society and the medical system respond to life-threatening illness. Clinicians deliver generally excellent technical medical care but often do a terrible job of meeting the human needs of patients and families. They can inadvertently damage the minds, souls, and bodies of the people under their care. I have argued that the advance directive, the device that has been the default solution to many of these problems, is deeply flawed, though some early glimmers of hope may soon bear fruit. I have also added my own voice and experience regarding possible ways forward. All these improvements will take time, energy, and money. Before the research can be done and reforms implemented, a lot of people will be admitted to intensive care units that operate in the old way.

So a valid question is, What should we do in the meanwhile? What should clinicians, who will one day be patients themselves, do? What should we all do in society? Do we fill out a living will with our attorney just in case? Is there a manual we should bring with us to the hospital? Should we be lobbying for changes in legislation?

In this epilogue I lay out how I plan to deal with these problems for myself and my family, for now.

Start by thinking about who will be walking the valley of shadows with you when you get sick or otherwise appear to be starting the transition from life to death. This may be a spouse, a child, a friend, a neighbor, or a person referred from a church or government office. Decide who that person will be and let them know that you would like them to speak for you if you should ever lose the ability to speak for yourself. It would be reasonable to complete a "durable power of attorney for healthcare" document that names this person as your proxy decision maker, especially if it's someone other than your legal spouse.

Write that person a Not Left Unsaid letter or have "the conversation" with him or her. Focus not so much on the grisly details of your hypothetical death but on what you love about life, about that person, and about your life together. Use Byock's Four Things or an equivalent to get the letter or conversation started. This step is important for two main reasons. Evidence suggests that family members with unresolved conflicts with the patient are the most likely to make decisions that leave everyone worse off. Since life's meaning is in our relationships, we should allow the shadow cast by our inevitable mortality to strengthen those relationships. There is no escaping that shadow, so we ought to use it for our benefit. It's more important, in my view, to be square with the people you love than it is to hammer out the speculative details about a permanent vegetative state you'll almost certainly never enter.

I've watched enough of these encounters to think that it's helpful to limit the melodrama so that people aren't afraid to talk to you about possibly relevant medical issues. But in any case, make sure that something beautiful comes from the consideration of difficult topics together.

Have a conversation about your sensibilities about medical treatments when life may be near its end. If my Five Approaches seem useful, use those. If they don't, it's probably not worth the stress of trying to map your ideas onto specific treatment programs at this point in time. Most people prefer intensive treatment unless it has reached the point of absurdity. If you're in the small minority that wants treatment beyond that point, say to maintain you in a permanent vegetative state, you should let your spokesperson know that. Otherwise, let them know your general philosophy about the role of medical treatments in life's wrapping-up scenes. Throughout the process, remember that your death will be at least partly in vain if the specter of mortality has not made your life richer while you still have it to enjoy.

When you reach a point where you feel like your life is starting to wind up, have the conversation again. It will probably be more emotional this time because the possibility of your death will be more real. But having had the conversation earlier will make it a little easier to have it again. After having the conversation again, schedule a consultation with a geriatrician or a palliative care physician. They are the people who, in the current medical system, are most likely to be attuned to the human side of life's final stages. They are the key practitioners of "slow medicine." They may be able to help you navigate new medical problems and possible operations or hospitalizations. If you have a trusted physician of long standing, it's reasonable to talk with them first. You could easily use your annual physical (or equivalent) to ask, "Would you be surprised if I were to die in the next five years?" When her answer becomes "No," that will be an indication that it's worth having the conversation and making additional plans. For a major conversation with a physician, particularly the geriatrician or palliative care physician, bring your spokesperson with you, so that everyone understands and remembers together.

When the time comes for you to be admitted to the hospital, ask to speak with the senior physician providing your care and tell him or her that you want to be treated as a whole person and describe how you like to communicate about important topics. Explain that you are aware that sometimes it's difficult to talk about the possibility that a treatment won't work, but that you are prepared to have an honest and full conversation. It may help to remind them that the current system of "code status" and "living wills" doesn't really deal with the complexity and uncertainty in any given illness, so you're not asking for something that simplistic. They may also need a reminder that right now most people who claim to be DNR or DNI are just trying to avoid the permanent vegetative state.

It's reasonable to undertake the first two steps now, whatever your age. There is healing in them, and it's always helpful to have a medical spokesperson. It's probably okay to wait to start the rest of the process until you hit sixty-five or seventy or develop a chronic medical illness like heart failure, adult diabetes, kidney failure, or emphysema. It's not that you should be afraid to live in some awareness of your own mortality, but the specific details of medical care aren't terribly relevant to you at an earlier phase of life. Live with a gentle awareness of mortality, but don't obsess about the medical questions until there's a significant chance they will actually matter.

Notice that I haven't suggested completing a living will. They just aren't useful in their current forms except perhaps as tokens to persuade people to have conversations. There are a few exceptions to my general objection to living wills. If your family members are hopelessly contentious and you know that they will be fighting with each other if you are ever lying unconscious in an ICU bed, a living will might help. If you worry that the medical system will not respect your family situation (e.g., you are not married to your life partner or you are socially stigmatized for some reason), they may make sense too. In those cases, the Make Your Wishes Known program might be of some use. Typical living wills generally are not.

Whatever you decide and however you implement your decisions, I would ask you to do two things. Live life as fully as you can, allowing occasional brushes with mortality to fill your life with meaning. And do not let your physicians and nurses or the system in which they operate fail you as a person. Demand the treatment you deserve as a human being, always.

NOTES

Introduction

1. Daniel Callahan, *The Troubled Dream of Life: In Search of a Peaceful Death* (Washington: Georgetown University Press, 2000), 180, 191–95.
2. Stacy's story is extensively hybridized.
3. I agree on this point with Tonelli MR, Misak CJ. Compromised autonomy and the seriously ill patient. *Chest* 2010;137:926–31.
4. Tidemalm D, et al. Risk of suicide after suicide attempt according to coexisting psychiatric disorder: Swedish cohort study with long term follow-up. *British Medical Journal* 2008;337:a2205. See also Brown SM, et al. Withdrawal of Nonfutile Life Support after Attempted Suicide. *American Journal of Bioethics* 2013;13(3):3–12.
5. Brown SM, Rozenblum R, Aboumatar H, et al. Defining patient and family engagement in the intensive care unit. *Am J Respir Crit Care Med* 2015;191:358–60.

Chapter 1

1. Peter Metcalf and Richard Huntington, *Celebrations of Death: The Anthropology of Mortuary Ritual*, 2nd ed., revised (Cambridge: Cambridge University Press, 1991).
2. Key books on this topic include Philippe Aries, *The Hour of Our Death* (New York: Alfred Knopf, 1981) and Drew Gilpin Faust, *This Republic of Suffering: Death and the American Civil War* (New York: Knopf, 2008).

3. The classic exposition of the changes in prestige and authority for physicians is Paul Starr, *The Social Transformation of American Medicine* (New York: Basic Books, 1982).

4. James Farrell, *Inventing the American Way of Death, 1830–1920* (Philadelphia: Temple University Press, 1980).

5. Lou Taylor, *Mourning Dress: A Costume and Social History* (New York: Routledge, 2009) describes this history in England; the situation in American cities was similar in relevant respects.

6. The demographic transition also involves changes in fertility. See Greenwood J, Seshadri A. The U.S. demographic transition. *American Economic Review* 2002;92(2):153–59, and Olshansky SJ, Ault AB. The fourth stage of the epidemiologic transition: the age of delayed degenerative diseases. *Milbank Quarterly* 2986;64(3):355–91.

7. Cosgrove J. The McKeown thesis: a historical controversy and its enduring influence. *American Journal of Public Health* 2002;92(5):725–29.

8. Bureau of the Census, *Historical Statistics of the United States 1789–1945* (Washington, DC: Bureau of the Census, 1949), 45.

9. Emily K. Abel, *The Inevitable Hour: A History of Caring for Dying Patients in America* (Baltimore, MD: Johns Hopkins University Press, 2013).

10. Hui D, et al. Clinical signs of impending death in cancer patients. *Oncologist* 2014;19(6):681–87.

11. Deep breaths can circulate blood, at least for a time. This phenomenon allows people in electrophysiology labs to maintain a pulse by coughing rhythmically while their heart fibrillates, unable to circulate blood on its own, during a procedure.

12. Oliver Wendell Holmes, *Currents and Cross-Currents in Medical Science: An Address Delivered before the Massachusetts Medical Society at the Annual Meeting, May 30, 1860* (Boston: Ticknor and Fields, 1860), 38.

13. David Rothman, *Strangers at the Bedside: A History Of How Law And Bioethics Transformed Medical Decision Making* (New York: Basic Books, 1992), 156–59, 165–67, argues that heart transplant played a crucial role in the cultural changes within medicine from 1967 to 1977.

14. Hilberman M. The evolution of intensive care units. *Crit Care Med* 1975;3:159–65.

15. Hilberman, "Evolution."

16. There were rare dangerous reactions to anesthesia or occasional good luck where no electricity was required. Electricity is now a mainstay of advanced cardiac life support.

17. Beck CS, et al. Ventricular fibrillation of long duration abolished by electric shock. *JAMA* 1947;135(15): 985–86. This in his own operating room, after a 1939 editorial browbeating colleagues for not having "resuscitation squads" ready to provide electrical shocks at a moment's notice.

18. Zoll P, et al. Termination of ventricular fibrillation in man by externally applied electric countershock. *New England Journal of Medicine* 1956;254(16):727–32, and Zoll P, et al. Ventricular fibrillation: treatment and prevention by external electric currents. *New England Journal of Medicine* 1960;262(3):105–12. We still call the adhesive electrical pads used to perform the procedure Zoll Pads.

19. Paracelsus (1493–1541) was an alchemist and physician, while Vesalius (1514–1564) was a founder of modern anatomy.

20. These were general variants of the enema or "clyster" techniques. See, e.g., Hughes JT. Miraculous deliverance of Anne Green: an Oxford case of resuscitation in the seventeenth century. *British Medical Journal* 1982;285:1792–93. On other creative uses of enemas, see James Whorton, *Inner Hygiene: Constipation and the Pursuit of Health in Modern Society* (New York: Oxford University Press, 2000).

21. West JB. The physiological challenges of the 1952 Copenhagen poliomyelitis epidemic and a renaissance in clinical respiratory physiology. *J Appl Physiol (1985)* 2005;99(2):424–32, provides a useful if somewhat technical overview.

22. Cresci G, Mellinger J. The history of nonsurgical enteral tube feeding access. *Nutr Clin Pract* 2006;21:522. The force-feeding of inmates observed in association with the twenty-first-century "War on Terror" has, in retrospect, a long and tangled history.

23. This is a fundamental argument of Rothman, *Strangers at the Bedside*.

24. Symmers WS. Not allowed to die. *British Medical Journal* 1968;1(5589): 442.

25. Starr, *Social Transformation of American Medicine* is the standard history of this process.

26. The best-known of many was New York's La Guardia Hospital: Rothman, *Strangers at the Bedside*, 235–37.

27. Mark Lytle, *America's Uncivil Wars* (New York: Oxford University Press, 2005).

28. While he does not use the precise framing of "aristocracy," Rothman, in *Strangers at the Bedside*, makes a version of this argument at length.

29. See especially, Aries's influential *The Hour of Our Death*.

30. For more on Saunders, see Milton Lewis, *Medicine and Care of the Dying: A Modern History* (New York: Oxford University Press, 2006).

31. Jessica Mitford, *The American Way of Death* (New York: Simon and Schuster, 1963).

Chapter 2

1. *The Milwaukee Sentinel*, April 2, 1973, page 4. See the contemporary discussion in David Dempsey, "The Living Will," *New York Times Magazine*, June 23, 1974, 12–13, 20–23.

2. Pope John Paul II. On life-sustaining treatments and the vegetative state: scientific advances and ethical dilemmas. *National Catholic Bioethics Quarterly* 2004;4(3):573–76. The Pope argued that tube feeding should be considered obligatory and had a strong influence on the thinking of many religious conservatives.

3. This connection between abortion and controversial life support therapy is remarkably consistent. See, e.g., Ronald Dworkin, *Life's Dominion: An Argument About Abortion, Euthanasia, and Individual Freedom* (New York: Knopf, 1993).

4. Dworkin, *Life's Dominion*, analyzes this notion of context in terms of critical goods associated with the overall shape of one's life but doesn't engage the question of narrative framing. There is of course a cognitive bias that emphasizes how events or experiences end, differentially weighting final as opposed to nonfinal events.

5. Dan Brock and Margaret Pabst Battin are two of the best-known proponents of the lack of a distinction between killing and letting die. Brock's relevant works are collected in *Life and Death: Philosophical Essays in Biomedical Ethics* (Cambridge: Cambridge University Press, 1993). Battin's main books on the topic are *The Least Worst Death: Essays in Bioethics on the End of Life* (New York: Oxford University Press, 1994) and *Ending Life: Ethics and the Way We Die* (New York: Oxford University Press, 2005). An important early essay on this question was Rachels J. Active and passive euthanasia. *N Engl J Med* 1975;292:78–80.

6. Norman Cantor, *Advance Directives and the Pursuit of Death with Dignity* (Bloomington, IN: Indiana University Press, 1993), preferred "prospective" autonomy, but "precedent" is more common in the literature and, I believe, more straightforwardly communicates what is happening with these determinations about hypothetical futures.

7. Allen Buchanan and Dan Brock, *Deciding for Others: The Ethics of Surrogate Decision Making* (Cambridge: Cambridge University Press, 1990), Chapter 2.

8. Suhl J, Simons P, Reedy T, Garrick T. Myth of substituted judgment: surrogate decision making regarding life support is unreliable. *Arch Intern Med* 1994;154:90–96; Shalowitz DI, et al. The accuracy of surrogate decision makers: a systematic review. *Arch Intern Med* 2006;166:493–97; Seckler AB, et al. Substituted judgment: how accurate are proxy predictions? *Ann Intern Med* 1991;115(2):92–98; Uhlmann RF, et al. Physicians' and spouses' predictions of elderly patients' resuscitation preferences. *J Gerontol* 1988;43(5):M115–21; White DB, Malvar G, Karr J, et al. Expanding the paradigm of the physician's role in surrogate decision-making: an empirically derived framework. *Crit Care Med* 2010;38(3):743–50; Scheunemann LP, Arnold RM, White

DB. The facilitated values history: helping surrogates make authentic decisions for incapacitated patients with advanced illness. *Am J Respir Crit Care Med* 2012;186(6):480–86.

9. Puchalski CM, et al. Patients who want their family and physician to make resuscitation decisions for them: observations from SUPPORT and HELP. Study to Understand Prognoses and Preferences for Outcomes and Risks of Treatment. Hospitalized Elderly Longitudinal Project. *J Am Geriatr Soc* 2000;48(5 Suppl):S84–90; Hawkins NA, et al. Micromanaging death: process preferences, values, and goals in end-of-life medical decision making. *Gerontologist* 2005;45(1):107–17; Fagerlin A, Ditto PH, Danks JH, et al. Projection in surrogate decisions about life-sustaining medical treatments. *Health Psychology* 2001;20:166–75.

10. Wendler D, Rid A. Systematic review: the effect on surrogates of making treatment decisions for others. *Ann Intern Med* 2011;154:336–46, summarizes the evidence.

11. Proponents of the pioneering California Natural Death act sometimes argued that living wills (as opposed to simple proxy documents) were to protect people from family members who might propose decisions "disturbed by grief, guilt and sometimes greed." California's Natural Death Act-Medical Staff Conference. University of California, San Francisco. *West J Med* 1978;128:318–30, 324.

12. California's Natural Death Act-Medical Staff Conference.

13. See Ben-Shahar and Schneider, *More Than You Wanted to Know* (Princeton, NJ: Princeton University Press, 2014).

14. Ben-Shahar and Schneider, in *More Than You Wanted to Know*, review this literature at length.

15. For another example of an extremely detailed living will, see Moroni Leash, *Strengthening Advance Directives: Overcoming Past Limitations through Enhanced Theory, Design, and Application* (Las Vegas: Lifecare, 2009).

16. Ceci Conolly, "President Gets Personal at Forum on Health Care," *Washington Post*, July 29, 2009.

17. Hickman SE, Sabatino CP, Moss AH, Nester JW. The POLST (Physician Orders for Life-Sustaining Treatment) paradigm to improve end-of-life care: potential state legal barriers to implementation. *J Law Med Ethics* 2008;36:119–40, 4.

18. Cosgriff JA, Pisani M, Bradley EH, et al. The association between treatment preferences and trajectories of care at the end-of-life. *J Gen Intern Med* 2007;22:1566–71.

19. Luce J. A history of resolving conflicts over end-of-life care in intensive care units in the United States. *Crit Care Med* 2010;38:1623–29. Luce reviews the history of debates about futility. See also Helft PR, et al. The rise and fall of the futility movement. *N Engl J Med* 2000;343(4):293–96.

20. See, for instance, Burns JP, Truog RD. Futility: A concept in evolution. *Chest* 2007;132(6):1987–93. The most recent consideration of the problem framed the issue as "potentially inappropriate" rather than "futile" care to recognize the problems with futility per se: Bosslet GT, Pope TM, Rubenfeld GD, et al. An Official ATS/AACN/ACCP/ESICM/ SCCM Policy Statement: Responding to Requests for Potentially Inappropriate Treatments in Intensive Care Units. *Am J Respir Crit Care Med* 2015;191(11):1318–1330.

21. See the lucid response of Neuberg GW. The cost of end-of-life care: a new efficiency measure falls short of AHA/ACC standards. *Circ Cardiovasc Qual Outcomes* 2009;2:127–33.

22. Emanuel EJ, et al. The economics of dying: the illusion of cost savings at the end of life. *N Engl J Med* 1994;330(8):540–44. Also, Teno J, et al. The illusion of end-of-life resource savings with advance directives: Support investigators. Study to Understand Prognoses and Preferences for Outcomes and Risks of Treatment. *J Am Geriatr Soc* 1997;45(4):513–18.

23. Schneiderman LJ, Kronick R, Kaplan RM, et al. Effects of offering advance directives on medical treatments and costs. *Ann Intern Med* 1992;117:599–606.

24. Gawande, *Being Mortal: Medicine and What Matters in the End* (New York: Metropolitan Books, 2014), 73–77, 92–95.

25. The Italians, originators of the Slow Food movement, have played an important role in Slow Medicine, which remains very much a work in progress. See, e.g., Vernero S, et al. Italy's "Doing more does not mean doing better" campaign. *BMJ* 2014;349:g4703.

26. Committee on Approaching Death, *Dying in America: Improving Quality and Honoring Individual Preferences Near the End of Life* (National Academies Press, 2014). Their first report, *Approaching Death*, came in 1997.

27. Jennett B, Plum F. Persistent vegetative state after brain damage. *Lancet* 1972;1(7753):734–37. The terminology of "permanent vegetative state" came later, as a way to refer to a persistent vegetative state that no longer appeared reversible.

28. Bryan Jennett, *The Vegetative State: Medical Facts, Ethical and Legal Dilemmas* (Cambridge: Cambridge University Press, 2002), 57–64.

Chapter 3

1. On Schiavo, see Lois Shepherd, *If That Ever Happens to Me: Making Life and Death Decisions after Terri Schiavo* (Chapel Hill: University of North Carolina Press, 2009).

2. Jay Katz, *The Silent World of Doctor and Patient* (New York: The Free Press, 1984), 123–25; Jodi Halpern, *From Detached Concern to Empathy: Humanizing Medical Practice* (New York: Oxford University Press, 2001).

3. Sudore RL, Fried TR. Redefining the "planning" in advance care planning: preparing for end-of-life decision making. *Ann Intern Med* 2010;153:256–61, makes a similar argument.

4. Buchanan and Brock, *Deciding for Others*, 50–57.

5. Charles Taylor wrote an influential treatment of authenticity as a view on modernism: *The Ethics of Authenticity* (Cambridge, MA: Harvard University Press, 1992). I am not using the term in Taylor's sense here.

6. Gerald Dworkin defines autonomy as, roughly, authenticity plus independence. I agree with him in broad terms; my worry about the current autonomism is that it has focused on a kind of superficial independence that saps autonomy of authenticity. See Dworkin G. Autonomy and behavior control. *Hastings Cent Rep* 1976;6:23–28.

7. Pope TM. Counting the dragon's teeth and claws: the definition of hard paternalism. *Ga State Univ Law Rev* 2004;20:659–722. The bridge example comes from chapter 5 of Mill's *On Liberty*.

8. Halpern, *Empathy*.

9. Schonwetter RS, Walker RM, Solomon M, et al. Life values, resuscitation preferences, and the applicability of living wills in an older population. *J American Geriatrics Society* 1996;44:954–58.

10. Puchalski CM, et al. "Patients who want their family and physician to make resuscitation decisions for them," and Hawkins NA, et al. "Micromanaging death."

11. This is the claim of Buchanan and Brock, *Deciding for Others*, 115–17.

12. Buchanan and Brock, *Deciding for Others*, 96–117, especially 115–16.

13. Ben-Shahar and Schneider, *More Than You Wanted to Know*, review these data at length.

14. Teno JM, Stevens M, Spernak S, Lynn J. Role of written advance directives in decision making: insights from qualitative and quantitative data. *J Gen Intern Med* 1998;13:439–46.

15. Mueller LA, Reid KI, Mueller PS. Readability of state-sponsored advance directive forms in the United States: a cross sectional study. *BMC Med Ethics* 2010;11:6.

16. Hoffmann DE, et al. The dangers of directives or the false security of forms. *J. Law. Med. Ethics.* 1996;24(1):11–13.

17. Jesus J, et al. Preferences for resuscitation and intubation among patients with do-not-resuscitate/do-not-intubate orders. *Mayo Clinic Proceedings* 2013;88(7):658–65. See also the similar findings from Connecticut a decade earlier: Upadya A, et al. Patient, physician, and family member understanding of living wills. *Am J Respir Crit Care Med* 2002;166(11):1430–35.

18. In re Hanford L. Pinette, No. 48-2004-MH-1519-O (Fla Cir Ct Orange Cty Nov 23, 2004), documents supplied by the court and in author's possession. Incidentally, the publicly available court documents do not obviously identify Hank as anything but chronically critically ill, a serious condition that about a third of patients ultimately survive. It is therefore not even clear that his living will literally applied, given the "no medical probability" of recovery enshrined by Florida living wills at the time.

19. I agree with Shepherd, *After Terri Schiavo*, 117, on this point.

20. See Robert Putnam and David Campbell, *American Grace: How Religion Divides and Unites Us* (New York: Simon and Schuster, 2012). Specifically as it relates to treatment near the end of life, see Torke AM, Garas NS, Sexson W, Branch WT. Medical care at the end of life: views of African American patients in an urban hospital. *J Palliat Med* 2005;8(3):593–602.

21. Muni S, Engelberg RA, Treece PD, et al. The influence of race/ethnicity and socioeconomic status on end-of-life care in the ICU. *Chest* 2011;139:1025–33.

22. Albaeni A, Chandra-Strobos N, Vaidya D, Eid SM. Predictors of early care withdrawal following out-of-hospital cardiac arrest. *Resuscitation* 2014;85(11):1455–61.

23. Rhondali W, Perez-Cruz P, Hui D, et al. Patient-physician communication about code status preferences: a randomized controlled trial. *Cancer* 2013;119(11):2067–73.

24. Upadya A, et al. "Patient, physician, and family member understanding of living wills"; Waite KR, Federman AD, McCarthy DM, et al. Literacy and race as risk factors for low rates of advance directives in older adults. *J Am Geriatr Soc* 2013;61(3):403–406. As a reminder that people of color are highly diverse, Asians tend in general to be more like Whites when it comes to advance directives: Gutierrez C, Hsu W, Ouyang Q, et al. Palliative care intervention in the intensive care unit: comparing outcomes among seriously ill Asian patients and those of other ethnicities. *J Palliat Care.* 2014;30(3):151–57.

25. West SK, Hollis M. Barriers to completion of advance care directives among African Americans ages 25–84: a cross-generational study. *Omega* (Westport). 2012;65(2):125–37; Melhado L, Bushy A. Exploring uncertainty in advance care planning in African Americans: does low health literacy influence decision making preference at end of life? *Am J Hosp Palliat Care* 2011;28(7):495–500.

26. Caralis PV, Davis B, Wright K, Marcial E. The influence of ethnicity and race on attitudes toward advance directives, life-prolonging treatments, and euthanasia. *J Clin Ethics* 1993;4:155–65; Wenger NS, Pearson ML, Desmond KA, et al. Epidemiology of do-not-resuscitate orders: disparity

by age, diagnosis, gender, race, and functional impairment. *Arch Intern Med* 1995;155:2056–62.

27. See http://www.pewforum.org/2013/11/21/views-on-end-of-life-medical-treatments/.

28. Caralis PV, et al., "The influence of ethnicity and race," 157.

29. Blackhall LJ, Frank G, Murphy ST, et al. Ethnicity and attitudes towards life sustaining technology. *Soc Sci Med* 1999;48(12):1779–89.

30. Caralis PV, et al. "The influence of ethnicity and race," 157.

31. Welch LC, Teno JM, Mor V. End-of-life care in black and white: race matters for medical care of dying patients and their families. *J Am Geriatr Soc* 2005;53:1145–53; Loggers ET, Maciejewski PK, Paulk E, et al. Racial differences in predictors of intensive end-of-life care in patients with advanced cancer. *J Clin Oncol* 2009;27:5559–64.

32. Gruneir A, Mor V, Weitzen S, et al. Where people die: a multilevel approach to understanding influences on site of death in America. *Med Care Res Rev* 2007;64:351–78.

33. Perkins HS, Geppert CM, Gonzales A, et al. Cross-cultural similarities and differences in attitudes about advance care planning. *J Gen Intern Med* 2002;17:48–57.

34. Bryan Jennett, *The Vegetative State: Medical Facts, Ethical and Legal Dilemmas* (Cambridge: Cambridge University Press, 2002), 36–41, based on his probably inflated estimate of 17 incident annual cases per million population.

35. Teno JM, Licks S, Lynn J, et al. Do advance directives provide instructions that direct care? SUPPORT Investigators. Study to Understand Prognoses and Preferences for Outcomes and Risks of Treatment. *J Am Geriatr Soc* 1997;45:508–12.

36. Hartog CS, Peschel I, Schwarzkopf D, et al. Are written advance directives helpful to guide end-of-life therapy in the intensive care unit? A retrospective matched-cohort study. *J Crit Care* 2014;29(1):128–33.

37. About 90 percent of deaths in modern American ICUs are negotiated, according to data from a period in which advance directives were rare. Prendergast TJ, et al. Increasing incidence of withholding and withdrawal of life support from the critically ill. *Am J Respir Crit Care Med* 1997;155(1):15–20.

38. Knaus W. APACHE 1978–2001: The development of a quality assurance system based on prognosis: milestones and personal reflections. *Archives of Surgery* 2002;137:37–41.

39. Knaus WA, Zimmerman JE, Wagner DP, et al. APACHE-Acute Physiology and Chronic Health Evaluation: a physiologically based classification system. *Crit Care Med* 1981;9:591–97.

40. Knaus WA, et al. Short-term mortality predictions for critically ill hospitalized adults: science and ethics. *Science* 1991;254(5030):389–94. Compare

Luce JM, Wachter RM. The ethical appropriateness of using prognostic scoring systems in clinical management. *Crit Care Clin* 1994;10:229–41.

41. Bayesianists protest that they have an appropriate response to this question, although theirs is more an expression of philosophical conviction than an accurate scientific response. Richard Jeffrey, *Subjective Probability: The Real Thing* (Cambridge, UK: Cambridge University Press, 2004) provides an engaging if rather technical overview of applied Bayesianist philosophy.

42. For the skeptics, consider that models with an area under the curve of 0.75 are routinely published. I have done it myself. Such models may be useful for benchmarking and hypothesis generation, but they are *not* useful for individual prediction. Ware J. The limitations of risk factors as prognostic tools. *N Engl J Med* 2006;355:2615–17, provides a useful discussion of this point.

43. Commonly, statisticians measure the usefulness ("calibration," the measure most relevant to patient-level decision-making) of prediction scores in terms of how well they perform in blocks of 10 percent ("deciles") of the population. Within that given decile the average predicted risk is compared to the observed mortality. With the sophisticated APACHE IV model, the 10 percent of patients with the highest risk of death have an average risk of death of 63 percent. It is not very reassuring for a score that the very sickest 10 percent of patients have almost a 50–50 chance of survival.

44. Lynn J, Harrell F, Jr., Cohn F, et al. Prognoses of seriously ill hospitalized patients on the days before death: implications for patient care and public policy. *New Horiz* 1997;5:56–61.

45. Keegan MT, et al. Severity of illness scoring systems in the intensive care unit. *Crit Care Med* 2011;39(1):163–69.

46. Redelmeier DA, Tversky A. Discrepancy between medical decisions for individual patients and for groups. *N Engl J Med* 1990;322(16):1162–64.

47. On hindsight bias, see Richard Thaler's *Misbehaving: The Making of Behavioral Economics* (New York: Norton, 2015), chapter 3.

48. Rocker G, et al. Clinician predictions of intensive care unit mortality. *Crit Care Med* 2004;32(5):1149–54.

49. McClish DK, Powell SH. How well can physicians estimate mortality in a medical intensive care unit? *Med. Decis. Making.* 1989;9(2):125–32. See similar studies in Poses RM, et al. The answer to "What are my chances, doctor?" depends on whom is asked: prognostic disagreement and inaccuracy for critically ill patients. *Crit Care Med* 1989;17(8):827–33 and Christensen C, et al. Forecasting survival in the medical intensive care unit: a comparison of clinical prognoses with formal estimates. *Methods Inf Med* 1993;32(4):302–308.

50. Lynn J, et al. Prognoses of Seriously Ill Hospitalized Patients on the Days before Death: Implications for Patient Care and Public Policy. *New Horizons* 1997;5(1):56–61.

51. Sinuff T, et al. Mortality predictions in the intensive care unit: comparing physicians with scoring systems. *Critical Care Medicine* 2006;34(3):878–85. Two other studies showed physicians performed a little better than the score, although neither worked as well as advance directives would require: Brannen AL, 2nd, Godfrey LJ, Goetter WE. Prediction of outcome from critical illness: a comparison of clinical judgment with a prediction rule. *Arch Intern Med* 1989;149:1083–86; Meyer AA, Messick WJ, Young P, et al. Prospective comparison of clinical judgment and APACHE II score in predicting the outcome in critically ill surgical patients. *J Trauma* 1992;32:747–53.

52. Prendergast TJ, et al. "Increasing Incidence."

53. Samuel M. Brown, et al. Survival after shock requiring high-dose vasopressor therapy. *Chest* 2013;143(3):664–71.

54. Meadow W, et al. Power and limitations of daily prognostications of death in the medical ICU for outcomes in the following 6 months. *Crit Care Med* 2014;42:2387–92.

55. Pratt CM, et al. Long-term outcomes after severe shock. *Shock* 2015;43:128–32.

56. Recounted in book 12 of *The Odyssey*.

57. Dresser R. Precommitment: A misguided strategy for securing death with dignity. *Texas Law Review* 2003;81:1823–47.

58. Ditto PH, Smucker WD, Danks JH, et al. Stability of older adults' preferences for life-sustaining medical treatment. *Health Psychol* 2003;22(6):605–15.

59. Lockhart LK, Ditto PH, Danks JH, et al. The stability of older adults' judgments of fates better and worse than death. *Death Stud* 2001;25:299–317.

60. For a philosophical treatment of the relevance of the difference between the time of decision and the time of its application, see the careful work of Jeff McMahan, *The Ethics of Killing: Problems at the Margins of Life* (New York: Oxford University Press, 2003), with some extended discussion in David DeGrazia, *Human Identity and Bioethics* (Cambridge, UK: Cambridge University Press, 2005).

61. Rothman, *Strangers*, 205–207.

62. Ditto PH, Danks JH, Smucker WD, et al. Advance directives as acts of communication: a randomized controlled trial. *Arch Intern Med* 2001;161:421–30.

63. Fagerlin A, Schneider CE. Enough: the failure of the living will. *Hastings Cent Rep* 2004;34:30–42; Perkins HS. Controlling death: the false promise of advance directives. *Ann Intern Med* 2007;147:51–57; Billings JA. The need for safeguards in advance care planning. *J Gen Intern Med* 2012;27:595–600.

64. Wenger N, Shugarman LR, Wilkinson A. Advance directives and advance care planning: Report to Congress, 2008 [online]. Available at http://

aspe.hhs.gov/daltcp/reports/2008/ADCongRpt.htm. Accessed March 26, 2015.

65. Detering KM, Hancock AD, Reade MC, Silvester W. The impact of advance care planning on end of life care in elderly patients: randomised controlled trial. *BMJ* 2010;340:c1345. They studied a modification of the Respecting Choices system that I discuss in chapter 7.

66. Silveira MJ, Kim SY, Langa KM. Advance directives and outcomes of surrogate decision making before death. *N Engl J Med* 2010;362:1211–18.

67. Gillick MR. Reversing the code status of advance directives? *N Engl J Med* 2010;362:1239–40.

68. Tolle SW, Tilden VP, Nelson CA, Dunn PM. A prospective study of the efficacy of the physician order form for life-sustaining treatment. *J Am Ger Soc* 1998;46:1097–102.

69. Mirarchi FL, Cammarata C, Zerkle SW, et al. TRIAD VII: do prehospital providers understand Physician Orders for Life-Sustaining Treatment documents? *J Patient Saf* 2015;11:9–17; Mirarchi FL, Doshi AA, Zerkle SW, Cooney TE. TRIAD VI: how well do emergency physicians understand Physicians Orders for Life Sustaining Treatment (POLST) forms? *J Patient Saf* 2015;11:1–8.

70. The POLST forms actually do make sense in a formal palliative care environment, for instance when a patient is already on hospice. What worries me the most about POLST forms is how rarely, if ever, they are associated with discussions about meaning near the end of life or life-completion tasks. I do not think POLST forms should be allowed without such discussions having occurred first.

Chapter 4

1. In animals, these tissues are the "silver skin"; humans have them just the same as other mammals, and doctors call them *fascia*, from the Latin for a band or bandage.

2. The standard popular introductions are Dan Ariely, *Predictably Irrational: The Hidden Forces That Shape Our Decisions* (New York: HarperCollins, 2008), and Daniel Kahneman, *Thinking, Fast and Slow* (New York: Farrar, Straus, Giroux, 2011). The standard introduction to behavioral solutions is Roger Thaler and Cass Sunstein, *Nudge: Improving Decisions about Health, Wealth, and Happiness* (New Haven, CT: Yale University Press, 2008). See also Thaler, *Misbehaving*.

3. The classic paper on the availability heuristic is Tversky A and Kahneman D, "Availability: A Heuristic for Judging Frequency and Probability," *Cognitive Psychology* 1973; 4, 207–32.

4. Tversky A, Kahneman D. Judgment under uncertainty: Heuristics and biases. *Science* 1974;185:1124–30.

5. The "false consensus" effect is, in my view, a subset of false coherence. See Ross L, et al. The false consensus effect: an egocentric bias in social perception and attribution processes. *J Exp Soc Psychol* 1977;13(3):279–301.

6. The "halo" effect is attributed to Thorndike EL. A constant error in psychological ratings. *J Applied Psychol* 1920;4(1):25–29. The parallel representativeness heuristic operates in a similar kind of way, distorting probabilities on the basis of how well they match a kind of ideal type. The classic paper on representativeness is Kahneman D and Tversky A. Subjective probability: a judgment of representativeness. *Cogn Psychol* 1972;3(3):430–54.

7. The term "confirmation bias" is attributed to Peter Wason: Wason PC. On the failure to eliminate hypotheses in a conceptual task. *Q J Exp Psychol* (Psychology Press) 1960;12(3):129–40, although the term refers to a variety of observations from antiquity to the present, without the specificity requisite to a scientific construct.

8. About 66 percent in one study were doing durably quite well: Pollard C, Kennedy P. A longitudinal analysis of emotional impact, coping strategies and post-traumatic psychological growth following spinal cord injury: a 10-year review. *Br J Health Psychol* 2007;12:347–62.

9. Gilbert's *Stumbling on Happiness* (New York: Knopf, 2006) is the standard introduction to this field, especially as it related to happiness. Loewenstein and others discuss "projection bias" in reasonably similar terms. See, e.g., Loewenstein G. Projection bias in medical decision making. *Med Decision Making* 2005;25:96–105.

10. Some observers, misapprehending what is actually happening, have called this adaptation "denial" rather than re-equilibration.

11. Purdy describes these experiences in a May 2011 TED talk (http://www.ted.com/talks/amy_purdy_living_beyond_limits) called "Living beyond Limits."

12. Robert Burt, *Death Is That Man Taking Names: Intersections of American Medicine Law, and Culture* (Oakland: University of California Press, 2004), 8–11.

13. The main website for the TMT movement is http://www.tmt.missouri.edu/index.html. Accessed February 17, 2014.

14. Atul Gawande provides a useful overview of Carstensen's theories in *Being Mortal*, 94–100.

15. Steinhauser KE, et al. Factors considered important at the end of life by patients, family, physicians, and other care providers. *JAMA* 2000; 284:2476–82, suggests that only about a third of people prioritized dying at home; other surveys have reported higher proportions, but essentially all have ignored the implicit disclaimer in respondents' minds.

16. Aries, *Hour of Our Death*.

17. Botti S, McGill A. When choosing is not deciding: the effect of perceived responsibility on satisfaction. *J Consumer Res* 2012;33:211–19.

18. Kristina Orfali and Sheena Iyengar have done the most interesting work on these topics. See, e.g., Botti S, et al. Tragic choices: autonomy and emotional responses to medical decisions. *J Consumer Res* 2009;36:337–52.

19. Multiple lines of analysis confirm the lack of desire people feel for the burden. See, e.g., Vig EK, et al. Surviving surrogate decision-making: what helps and hampers the experience of making medical decisions for others. *J Gen Intern Med* 2007;22(9):1274–79; Botti S, et al., "Tragic choices"; Orfali K, et al. Autonomy gone awry: a cross-cultural study of parents' experiences in neonatal intensive care units. *Theor Med Bioeth* 2004;25(4):329–65; Orfali K. Parental role in medical decision-making: fact or fiction? A comparative study of ethical dilemmas in French and American neonatal intensive care units. *Soc Sci Med* 2004;58(10):2009–22.

20. On the ways the "medical industrial complex" can affect decision making among older individuals, see Sharon Kaufman, *Ordinary Medicine: Extraordinay Treatments, Living Longer, and Where to Draw the Line* (Durham, NC: Duke University Press, 2015). I discuss the notion of "clinical crossroads" in Chapter 8.

21. See, e.g., Morrison WE. Is that all you got? *J Palliat Med* 2010;13:1384–85.

22. See, e.g., Girotra S, Nallamothu BK, Spertus JA, et al. Trends in survival after in-hospital cardiac arrest. *N Engl J Med* 2012;367(20):1912–20. For the most recent data, they cite about a 21 percent survival after in-hospital CPR, with about 30 percent of those experiencing neurological disability of some kind. This suggests that around 15 percent of individuals who undergo in-hospital CPR survive without neurological disability. About half of those with disability have only moderate disability. Among patients with cardiac arrest as the result of more difficult-to-treat rhythms, the most recent survival rates were 14 percent, with about half of them free from disability, suggesting 7 percent survival with satisfactory neurological outcome. Recent improvements in survival could reflect greater use of hospice and DNR/DNI orders, leading to fewer patients with very advanced disease undergoing CPR; the researchers could not answer that question on the basis of their study.

23. The NNT is just the inverse of the absolute risk reduction or, equivalently, 100 divided by the risk reduction. An absolute risk reduction of 14 percent represents an NNT of about 7 (100/14 = 6.7). An absolute risk reduction of 7 percent represents an NNT of about 14 (100/7 = 14.3).

24. On a longer view of consecration, we current clinicians have honed our treatments on prior generations of patients; without their sacrifice we would not have the incredible survival rates that we see now in the contemporary ICU.

25. Wilkinson DJ, Truog RD. The luck of the draw: physician-related variability in end-of-life decision-making in intensive care. *Intensive Care Med* 2013;39(6):1128–32; Garland A., et al. Physicians' influence over decisions to forego life support. *J Palliat Med* 2007;10(6):1298–305.

26. See Truog RD. Do-not-resuscitate orders in evolution: matching medical interventions with patient goals. *Crit Care Med* 2011;39(5):1213–14; Henneman EA, Baird B, Bellamy PE, et al. Effect of do-not-resuscitate orders on the nursing care of critically ill patients. *Am J Crit Care* 1994;3(6):467–72; Chen JL, Sosnov J, Lessard D, Goldberg RJ. Impact of do-not-resuscitation orders on quality of care performance measures in patients hospitalized with acute heart failure. *Am Heart J* 2008;156(1):78–84; Cohen RI, Lisker GN, Eichorn A, et al. The impact of do-not-resuscitate orders on triage decisions to a medical intensive care unit. *J Crit Care* 2009;24(2):311–15; Beach MC, Morrison RS. The effect of do-not-resuscitate orders on physician decision-making. *J Am Geriatr Soc* 2002;50:2057–61.

27. Halpern, *From Detached Concern to Empathy*, 29. See also Kvale J, Berg L, Groff JY, et al. Factors associated with residents' attitudes toward dying patients. *Fam Med* 1999;31(10):691–96; Gorman TE, Ahern SP, Wiseman J, et al. Residents' end-of-life decision making with adult hospitalized patients: a review of the literature. *Acad Med* 2005;80(7):622–33.

28. See, e.g., Singh H., et al. Understanding diagnostic errors in medicine: a lesson from aviation. *Qual Saf Health Care* 2006;15(3):159–64; Singh H., et al. Exploring situational awareness in diagnostic errors in primary care. *BMJ Qual Saf* 2012;21(1):30–38.

29. Kathryn Montgomery, *How Doctors Think: Clinical Judgment and the Practice of Medicine* (New York: Oxford University Press, 2006).

30. Croskerry P. Perspectives on diagnostic failure and patient safety. *Healthc Q* 2012;15:50–56.

31. Malcolm Gladwell, *Outliers: The Story of Success* (New York: Little, Brown, 2008).

32. Mulley AG, Trimble C, Elwyn G. Stop the silent misdiagnosis: patients' preferences matter. *BMJ* 2012;345:e6572.

33. I review these studies in chapter 3.

34. Nicholas Christakis has documented this phenomenon extensively. See especially his *Death Foretold: Prophecy and Prognosis in Medical Care* (Chicago: University of Chicago Press, 1999).

35. See especially Meltzer LS, Huckabay LM. Critical care nurses' perceptions of futile care and its effect on burnout. *Am J Crit Care* 2004;13(3):202–208 and Embriaco N, Papazian L, Kentish-Barnes N, et al. Burnout syndrome among critical care healthcare workers. *Curr Opin Crit Care* 2007;13(5):482–88.

36. There is some controversy about what the rule actually is and what scientific literature establishes it, but the "Dunning-Kruger effect" refers to the observation that novices tend to overrate their abilities and experts tend to underrate theirs.

37. While I have had to flesh out some details from memory, this story is in its essentials that of my grand father, Howard Arthur Morris (1919–2004).

38. This breathing pattern was famously described in 1818 by the Irish physician John Cheyne. Cheyne associated the pattern with heart failure, but the same kind of unstable breathing can happen when the brain has swollen to the point that blood no long circulates normally (indeed, in Cheyne's patient the breathing pattern appeared only after a large stroke in a patient with chronic heart failure; Cheyne probably made the wrong inference, although his observation was still useful). Cheyne J. A case of apoplexy in which the fleshy part of the heart was converted into fat. *Dublin Hospital Reports* 1818;2:216–23. Even independent of the confusion about the stroke, Cheyne misdiagnosed the main finding of his report (what we would now call an epicardial fat pad), but his description of the breathing pattern has become classic. We should all be so lucky as physician scientists!

Chapter 5

1. Burt, *Death Is That Man Taking Names*, discusses this problem at some length. See especially pp. 88–94, 104–105.

2. Mechanical assist devices for failing hearts have their own sets of clicks and whirs and anxieties, but I don't discuss them here.

3. See the calls to reform in Barr J, Fraser GL, Puntillo K, et al. Clinical practice guidelines for the management of pain, agitation, and delirium in adult patients in the intensive care unit. *Crit Care Med* 2013;41:263–306, and Hopkins RO, Spuhler VJ, Thomsen GE. Transforming ICU culture to facilitate early mobility. *Crit Care Clin* 2007;23:81–96.

4. This is not what the movies and television mean by "shock"; the problem is not that people are surprised or frightened, although they often are. It is that their blood pressure is dangerously low.

5. No one knows the true incidence of delusional memories of sexual assault among ICU patients. It's hard to know how to broach the topic with ICU survivors without causing new emotional stress. As I speak with other researchers in this area, though, the problem appears to be distressingly common.

6. The literature is mixed at best, and "confounding by indication" plays an important role. While many people in the field have abandoned the Valium-like medications ("benzodiazepines"), the few studies that have pitted them directly against newer medications have failed to demonstrate clear superiority. See, e.g., Jackson JC, Girard TD, Gordon

SM, et al. Long-term cognitive and psychological outcomes in the awakening and breathing controlled trial. *Am J Respir Crit Care Med* 2010;182:183–91; Pandharipande PP, Pun BT, Herr DL, et al. Effect of sedation with dexmedetomidine vs lorazepam on acute brain dysfunction in mechanically ventilated patients: the MENDS randomized controlled trial. *JAMA* 2007;298:2644–53; Jackson JC, Santoro MJ, Ely TM, et al. Improving patient care through the prism of psychology: application of Maslow's hierarchy to sedation, delirium, and early mobility in the intensive care unit. *J Crit Care* 2014;29:438–44; Frontera JA. Delirium and sedation in the ICU. *Neurocrit Care* 2011;14:463–74; Mirski MA, Lewin JJ, 3rd, Ledroux S, et al. Cognitive improvement during continuous sedation in critically ill, awake and responsive patients: the Acute Neurological ICU Sedation Trial (ANIST). *Intensive Care Med* 2010;36:1505–13.

7. Richard Griffiths and Christina Jones, eds. *Intensive Care Aftercare* (Oxford, UK: Butterworth-Heinemann, 2002), 27–35.

8. Incidentally, the reports associated with CPR do not seem to differ from the general delusions of ICU patients, other than perhaps references to tunnel vision. The most thorough catalog of delusional memories associated with CPR is in Parnia S, Spearpoint K, de Vos G, et al. AWARE—AWAreness during REsuscitation—a prospective study. *Resuscitation* 2014;85:1799–805.

9. Griffiths and Jones, *Intensive Care Aftercare*, 31.

10. Skirrow P, et al. The impact of current media events on hallucinatory content: the experience of the intensive care unit (ICU) patient. *Br J Clin Psychol* 2002;41(1):87–91.

11. Griffiths and Jones, *Intensive Care Aftercare*, 27–35.

12. Baile WF, Buckman R, Lenzi R, et al. SPIKES—A six-step protocol for delivering bad news: application to the patient with cancer. *Oncologist* 2000;5:302–11. See also Arnold RM, Back AL, Barnato AE, et al. The Critical Care Communication project: improving fellows' communication skills. *J Crit Care* 2015;30(2):250–54.

13. The technical name is hemophagocytosis lymphohistiocytosis; I use hemophagocytosis syndrome here because it reads more easily.

14. Callahan, *Troubled Dream of Life*, 198–203.

Chapter 6

1. Rich's story is extensively hybridized.

2. See Kahn JM, Le T, Angus DC, et al. The epidemiology of chronic critical illness in the United States. *Crit Care Med* 2015;43:282–87, and Nelson JE, Cox CE, Hope AA, Carson SS. Chronic critical illness. *Am J Respir Crit Care Med* 2010;182:446–54.

3. Iwashyna T. Survivorship will be the defining challenge of critical care in the 21st century. *Ann Int Med* 2010;153:204–205.

4. Jones C, Skirrow P, Griffiths RD, et al. Rehabilitation after critical illness: a randomized, controlled trial. *Crit Care Med* 2003;31(10):2456–61.

5. Herridge MS, et al. Functional disability 5 years after acute respiratory distress syndrome. *N Engl J Med* 2011;364(14):1293–304.

6. Needham and colleagues summarize key evidence and strategies in Parker A, Sricharoenchai T, Needham DM. Early rehabilitation in the intensive care unit: preventing physical and mental health impairments. *Curr Phys Med Rehabil Rep* 2013;1:307–14.

7. Because of the structure of the research, ALTOS has been published as several parallel studies. See especially Needham DM, Dinglas VD, Morris PE, et al. Physical and cognitive performance of acute lung injury patients one year after initial trophic vs full enteral feeding: EDEN trial follow-up. *Am J Respir Crit Care Med* 2013; 188(5):567–76, and Needham DM, Dinglas VD, Bienvenu OJ, et al. One year outcomes in patients with acute lung injury randomised to initial trophic or full enteral feeding: prospective follow-up of EDEN randomised trial. *BMJ* 2013;346:f1532.

8. Needham D, et al. Improving long-term outcomes after discharge from intensive care unit: report from a stakeholders' conference. *Crit Care Med* 2012;40(2):502–509.

9. See, e.g., Netzer G, Sullivan DR. Recognizing, naming, and measuring a family intensive care unit syndrome. *Ann Am Thorac Soc* 2014;11:435–41; Davidson JE, Jones C, Bienvenu OJ. Family response to critical illness: postintensive care syndrome-family. *Crit Care Med* 2012;40:618–24; and Schmidt M, Azoulay E. Having a loved one in the ICU: the forgotten family. *Curr Opin Crit Care* 2012;18:540–47.

10. Griffiths and Jones, *Intensive Care Aftercare*, 12.

11. Needham DM, et al. "One year outcomes."

12. Griffiths and Jones, *Intensive Care Aftercare*, 48–50.

13. Griffiths and Jones, *Intensive Care Aftercare*, 14–16, 53–58.

14. See, e.g., Misak CJ. ICU-acquired weakness: obstacles and interventions for rehabilitation. *Am J Respir Crit Care Med* 2011;183:845–46, for a compelling example of the difficulties associated with recovery.

15. Robert M. Sapolsky, *Why Zebras Don't Get Ulcers*, 3rd ed., (New York: Holt Paperbacks, 2004), is a useful introduction to stress physiology.

16. Jones C, et al. Memory, delusions, and the development of acute posttraumatic stress disorder-related symptoms after intensive care. *Crit Care Med* 2001;29(3):573–80; Jones C, et al. Precipitants of post-traumatic stress disorder following intensive care: a hypothesis generating study of diversity in care. *Intensive Care Med* 2007;33(6):978–85; Tedstone JE, et al. Posttraumatic stress disorder following medical illness and treatment. *Clin Psychol Rev* 2003;23(3):409–48.

17. Zisook S, et al. PTSD following bereavement. *Ann Clin Psychiatry* 1998;10(4):157–63; Vachon ML, et al. Predictors and correlates of adaptation to conjugal bereavement. *Am J Psychiatry* 1982;139(8):998–1002.
18. Lynn-McHale DJ, et al. Need satisfaction levels of family members of critical care patients and accuracy of nurses' perceptions. *Heart Lung* 1988;17(4):447–53. In exploratory studies, five of the ten most important themes for families in the ICU involve improved information: Davidson JE. Facilitated sensemaking: a strategy and new middle-range theory to support families of intensive care unit patients. *Crit Care Nurse* 2010;30(6):28–39.
19. Zettel-Watson L, et al. Actual and perceived gender differences in the accuracy of surrogate decisions about life-sustaining medical treatment among older spouses. *Death Stud* 2008;32(3):273–90; Zier LS, et al. Surrogate decision makers' interpretation of prognostic information: a mixed-methods study. *Ann Intern Med* 2012;156(5):360–66.
20. Carl Schneider, *The Practice of Autonomy: Patients, Doctors, and Medical Decisions* (New York: Oxford University Press, 1998). See also Azoulay E, Pochard F, Kentish-Barnes N, et al. Risk of post-traumatic stress symptoms in family members of intensive care unit patients. *Am J Respir Crit Care Med* 2005;171(9):987–994.
21. Larson CO, et al. The relationship between meeting patients' information needs and their satisfaction with hospital care and general health status outcomes. *Int J Qual Health Care* 1996;8(5):447–56; Osborn TR, et al. Identifying elements of ICU care that families report as important but unsatisfactory: decision-making, control, and ICU atmosphere. *Chest* 2012;142(5):1185–92; Hanson LC, et al. What is wrong with end-of-life care? Opinions of bereaved family members. *J Am Geriatr Soc* 1997;45(11):1339–44; Azoulay E, et al. Half the families of intensive care unit patients experience inadequate communication with physicians. *Crit Care Med* 2000;28(8):3044–49.
22. The Vanderbilt group maintains the excellent website, http://icudelirium.org, a clearinghouse of information relevant to the field.
23. Cuthbertson BH, Elders A, Hall S, et al. Mortality and quality of life in the five years after severe sepsis. *Crit Care* 2013;17:R70.
24. Pratt CM, et al, "Long-term outcomes after severe shock."
25. Turnbull AE, et al. A scenario-based, randomized trial of patient values and functional prognosis on intensivist intent to discuss withdrawing life support. *Crit Care Med* 2014;42(6):1455–62.
26. It is possible that the values were not relevant because the values were expressed in typical living-will style and physicians intuitively felt that their advice already incorporated the information present in such limited directives. Determining the relative contributions of different components will take further research; what is clear is that priming with PICS increases recommendations to stop life support in simulated decision-making.

Chapter 7

1. See, e.g., Prommer EE. Using the values-based history to fine-tune advance care planning for oncology patients. *J Cancer Educ* 2010;25:66–69.

2. This moderation has met with occasional criticism from more extreme vantage points, especially after the 2004 papal statement against stopping artificial nutrition and fluids. See, e.g., Furton EJ. A critique of the five wishes: comments in the light of a papal statement. *Ethics Medics* 2005;30(3):3–4.

3. Bernard Hammes, ed., *Having Your Own Say: Getting the Right Care When It Matters Most* (Atlanta, GA: Center for Health Transformation Press, 2012); Pecanac KE, Repenshek MF, Tennenbaum D, Hammes BJ. Respecting Choices(R) and advance directives in a diverse community. *J Palliat Med* 2014;17:282–87. The reported experience in Milwaukee was disappointing. While it appeared that proxies were named more frequently among certain patient groups, the overall effect was of no change in advance directives or compliance with instructions contained in the very few advance directives that actually provided instructions regarding treatment. The Australian experience is reported in Detering KM, Hancock AD, Reade MC, Silvester W. The impact of advance care planning on end of life care in elderly patients: randomised controlled trial. *BMJ* 2010;340:c1345.

4. Hammes B, Rooney B. Death and end-of-life planning in one midwestern community. *Arch Int Med* 1998;158:383–90. Note that proxy designations are primarily relevant when an individual does not want her family to decide for her, because families are the legal default decision makers when a proxy is missing. The authors did not report how often the proxy designation was actually needed.

5. Hammes BJ, Rooney BL, Gundrum JD. A comparative, retrospective, observational study of the prevalence, availability, and specificity of advance care plans in a county that implemented an advance care planning microsystem. *J Am Geriatr Soc* 2010;58:1249–55.

6. The evidence is reviewed at length in Ben-Shahar and Schneider, *More Than You Wanted to Know.*

7. Sudore R, Fried T. Redefining the "planning" in advance care planning: preparing for end-of-life decision making. *Ann Intern Med* 2010;153:256–61; Sudore RL, Knight SJ, McMahan RD, et al. A novel website to prepare diverse older adults for decision making and advance care planning: a pilot study. *J Pain Symptom Manage* 2014;47:674–86.

8. Angelo Volandes, *The Conversation: A Revolutionary Plan for End-of-Life Care* (New York: Bloomsbury, 2015), details the philosophy that has driven his efforts to develop advance care planning videos.

9. Billings JA. The need for safeguards in advance care planning. *J Gen Intern Med* 2012;27:597, correctly identifies these problems with the videos.

10. See, e.g., El-Jawahri A, Podgurski LM, Eichler AF, et al. Use of video to facilitate end-of-life discussions with patients with cancer: a randomized controlled trial. *J Clin Oncol* 2010;28:305–10, and McCannon JB, O'Donnell WJ, Thompson BT, et al. Augmenting communication and decision making in the intensive care unit with a cardiopulmonary resuscitation video decision support tool: a temporal intervention study. *J Palliat Med* 2012;15:1382–87.

11. Wilson ME, Krupa A, Hinds RF, et al. A video to improve patient and surrogate understanding of cardiopulmonary resuscitation choices in the ICU: a randomized controlled trial. *Crit Care Med* 2015;43:621–29.

12. Stacey D, Legare F, Col NF, et al. Decision aids for people facing health treatment or screening decisions. *Cochrane Database Syst Rev* 2014;1:CD001431.

13. In general, see Stacey D, et al. "Decision aids." For a perspective specific to the ICU, see Cox CE, et al. A universal decision support system: addressing the decision-making needs of patients, families, and clinicians in the setting of critical illness. *Am J Respir Crit Care Med* 2014;190:4:366–73.

14. https://decisionaid.ohri.ca/decaids.html.

15. Cox CE, Lewis CL, Hanson LC, et al. Development and pilot testing of a decision aid for surrogates of patients with prolonged mechanical ventilation. *Crit Care Med* 2012;40:2327–34.

16. Benjamin Levi, *Respecting Patient Autonomy* (Urbana: University of Illinois Press, 1999).

17. Green MJ, Schubart JR, Whitehead MM, et al. Advance care planning does not adversely affect hope or anxiety among patients with advanced cancer. *J Pain Sympt Manage* 2015;49(6):1088–96; Schubart JR, Levi BH, Camacho F, et al. Reliability of an interactive computer program for advance care planning. *J Palliat Med* 2012;15:637–42.

18. Elwyn G, O'Connor A, Stacey D, et al. Developing a quality criteria framework for patient decision aids: online international Delphi consensus process. *BMJ* 2006;333(7565):417. These authors have begun actively engaging these concerns.

19. Curtis JR, Treece PD, Nielsen EL, et al. Randomized Trial of Communication Facilitators to Reduce Family Distress and Intensity of End-of-life Care. *Am J Respir Crit Care Med* 2016.

20. McDonagh JR, Elliott TB, Engelberg RA, et al. Family satisfaction with family conferences about end-of-life care in the intensive care unit: increased proportion of family speech is associated with increased satisfaction. *Crit Care Med* 2004;32(7):1484–88.

21. Tony Back in Seattle and Bob Arnold in Pittsburgh developed OncoTalk, a remarkably robust and useful training program for oncologists. While

the studies of this intervention have mostly explored whether physicians in training remember what they were taught, there is reason to be optimistic about the direction that improved communication is taking us. They have recently extended the approach to IntensiveTalk for the ICU.

22. Wright AA, Zhang B, Ray A, et al. Associations between end-of-life discussions, patient mental health, medical care near death, and caregiver bereavement adjustment. *JAMA* 2008;300:1665–73.

23. Bernacki RE, Block SD. American College of Physicians High Value Care Task F. Communication about serious illness care goals: a review and synthesis of best practices. *JAMA Intern Med* 2014;174:1994–2003; Bernacki RE, Block SD. Serious illness communications checklist. *Virtual Mentor* 2013;15:1045–49.

24. Jeff's story is not deidentified in any way.

25. See http://patientfamilyengagement.org.

Chapter 8

1. While the e-mail, in my possession, is reproduced verbatim here, the story that follows is lightly hybridized to maintain privacy.

2. Hilde Lindemann Nelson and James Lindemann Nelson, *The Patient in the Family: An Ethics of Medicine and Families* (New York: Routledge, 1995), provides a useful overview of considerations for families in medicine.

3. My protest of this policy is in Brown S. We still lack patient centered visitation in intensive care units. *BMJ* 2015;350:h792.

4. Very rarely, a family member is so emotionally overwhelmed, that she or he is unable to be present in the room without creating a dangerous distraction from the medical tasks at hand. I'm mindful that such an exclusion could easily be overinterpreted to justify broadly exclusionary policies. In my experience, this is only true of perhaps 1 percent of family members.

5. See, e.g., Garrouste-Orgeas M, Coquet I, Perier A, et al. Impact of an intensive care unit diary on psychological distress in patients and relatives. *Crit Care Med* 2012;40:2033–40, and Backman CG, Walther SM. Use of a personal diary written in the ICU during critical illness. *Intensive Care Med* 2001;27:426–29.

6. Pope TM. The maladaptation of Miranda to advance directives: a critique of the implementation of the Patient Self-Determination Act. *Health Matrix Clevel* 1999;9:139–202.

7. This phrase is also used in the communication literature. See, e.g., Back AL, Arnold RM, Quill TE. Hope for the best, and prepare for the worst. *Ann Intern Med* 2003;138:439–43.

8. Ira Byock, *Dying Well: Peace and Possibilities at the End of Life* (New York: Riverhead, 1998).

9. Ira Byock, *The Four Things That Matter Most: A Book about Living* (New York: Free Press, 2004); Harvey Chochinov, *Dignity Therapy: Final Words for Final Days* (New York: Oxford University Press, 2012).

10. Sharon Kaufman, *Ordinary Medicine: Extraordinay Treatments, Living Longer, and Where to Draw the Line* (Durham, NC: Duke University Press, 2015) considers implantable cardiac defibrillators and kidney dialysis as two paradigmatic interventions that often represent clinical crossroads for older individuals.

11. One of the elements of the ABIM Choosing Wisely campaign for critical care (http://www.choosingwisely.org/doctor-patient-lists/critical-care-societies-collaborative-critical-care/) is offering people the option of a natural death whenever aggressive treatment is proposed.

12. Daniel Kahneman, "Experienced Utility and Objective Happiness: A Moment-Based Approach," in Kahneman and Tversky, eds., *Choices, Values, and Frames* (Cambridge, UK: Cambridge University Press, 2000), 673–92, describes a distinction between experience and memory of experience, which is relevant to this point, although this question of prospect versus retrospect involves substantially more themes than just the measurement of utility.

13. Lampert R, Hayes DL, Annas GJ, et al. HRS expert consensus statement on the management of cardiovascular implantable electronic devices (CIEDs) in patients nearing end of life or requesting withdrawal of therapy. *Heart Rhythm* 2010;7:1008–26.

14. The Gundersen Healthcare approach to advance care planning does appropriately respond to different stages of advance care planning, a crucial element of their system.

15. Walkey A, et al. Derivation and validation of 5-year risk for mechanical ventilation among community-dwelling adults: The Framingham-Intermountain Anticipating Life Support Study (FIALS). *J Am Ger Soc* 2015;63(10):2082–8.

16. Dexter PR, et al. Effectiveness of computer-generated reminders for increasing discussions about advance directives and completion of advance directive forms: a randomized, controlled trial. *Ann Intern Med* 1998;128(2):102–10.

17. See, e.g., Christopher De Bono, "An Exploration and Adaptation of Anton T. Boisen's Notion of the Psychiatric Chaplain in Responding to Current Issues in Clinical Chaplaincy," PhD dissertation, University of St. Michael's College, 2012.

18. Strictly speaking, *doula* is the feminine of the Greek word, but in English usage now, the term "doula" does not require that the individual be a woman. Following that usage, I use doula in a gender-neutral sense.

19. Doug White's group has proposed "family support specialist" as a very similar role. White DB, et al. Nurse-led intervention to improve surrogate decision making for patients with advanced critical illness. *Am J Crit Care* 2012;21(6):396–409.

20. Megory Anderson, *Sacred Dying: Creating Rituals for Embracing the End of Life* (New York: Da Capo, 2003) describes a variety of such rituals. Deborah Cook and colleagues in Canada evaluated an intervention aimed at personalizing death as a kind of complement to the rituals Anderson proposes: Cook D, Swinton M, Toledo F, et al. Personalizing Death in the Intensive Care Unit: The 3 Wishes Project: A Mixed-Methods Study. *Ann Intern Med* 2015; 163: 271-279.

21. On family presence at CPR, see Robinson SM, Mackenzie-Ross S, Campbell Hewson GL, et al. Psychological effect of witnessed resuscitation on bereaved relatives. *Lancet* 1998;352(9128):614–17; Jabre P, Belpomme V, Azoulay E, et al. Family presence during cardiopulmonary resuscitation. *N Engl J Med* 2013;368(11):1008–18; and MacLean SL, Guzzetta CE, White C, et al. Family presence during cardiopulmonary resuscitation and invasive procedures: practices of critical care and emergency nurses. *Am J Crit Care* 2003;12(3):246–57.

22. David Rieff, *Swimming in a Sea of Death* (New York: Simon and Schuster, 2008).

23. Byock, *Four Things*.

24. Gawande, *Being Mortal*, 73–77, 92–95.

25. A few researchers and activists have spoken about creating a system of advance directives that emphasizes goals for outcomes rather than decisions about specific procedures along the way. See, e.g., Truog RD. Do-not-resuscitate orders in evolution: matching medical interventions with patient goals. *Crit Care Med* 2011;39:1213–14; Winzelberg GS, Hanson LC, Tulsky JA. Beyond autonomy: diversifying end-of-life decision-making approaches to serve patients and families. *J Am Geriatr Soc* 2005;53:1046–50; and Truog RD, Waisel DB, Burns JP. DNR in the OR: a goal-directed approach. *Anesthesiology* 1999;90:289–95.

26. Vanpee D, Swine C. Scale of levels of care versus DNR orders. *J Med Ethics* 2004;30(4):351–52, proposes four levels—terminal, palliative, usual, and intensive—and a positive framing, although this is specific to frail elderly individuals.

27. See especially Dennis McCullough, *Your Mother, My Mother* (New York: Harper Perennial, 2009).

28. I follow Dan Callahan's perceptive analysis in *Troubled Dream of Life*, 191–95, on this point.

INDEX